Massive Rotator Cuff Tears

Lawrence V. Gulotta · Edward V. Craig

Editors

Massive Rotator Cuff Tears

Diagnosis and Management

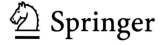 Springer

Editors
Lawrence V. Gulotta, MD
Sports Medicine and Shoulder Service
Hospital for Special Surgery
New York, NY, USA

Department of Orthopedic Surgery
Weill Cornell Medical School
New York, NY, USA

Edward V. Craig, MD, MPH
Professor of Clinical Surgery
Weill Cornell Medical School
New York, NY, USA

Attending Surgeon
Hospital for Special Surgery
New York, NY, USA

ISBN 978-1-4899-7493-8   ISBN 978-1-4899-7494-5 (eBook)
DOI 10.1007/978-1-4899-7494-5
Springer New York Heidelberg Dordrecht London

Library of Congress Control Number: 2014947468

Springer is part of Springer Science+Business Media (www.springer.com)

I dedicate this book to my wife, Megan, and my children for their support and encouragement. They make everything in my professional career possible.
I also dedicate this book to my patients. I have learned much from listening to them, and I look forward to learning more from them in the years to come.

Lawrence V. Gulotta, MD

This work is dedicated to my three daughters, Mackenzie, Kelsey, and Taylor, and to my wife Kathryn, collectively the foundation of my professional life—and the purpose of my personal one.

Edward V. Craig, MD

Preface

As the population ages and desires to remain active, we have seen a rise in the number of patients who present with chronic, massive rotator cuff tears. Perhaps a decade ago, we had very limited options for these patients and treatment decisions were made through more art than science. However, with the advent of the reverse shoulder arthroplasty, and a better understanding of the role of tendon transfers and arthroscopy, we now have sound options to offer these patients.

The goal of this book is to present a comprehensive approach to the patient with a massive rotator cuff tear. An overarching theme of the book is that patients with similar imaging findings may present with very different clinical presentations. Once the diagnosis of a massive rotator cuff tear is made, the final treatment recommendation should come down to the patient's main complaints and their expectations. We feel this book serves a unique, but quickly expanding, niche to guide the clinician through this challenging problem.

The book follows a logical path through the issues that surround massive rotator cuff tears. It begins with chapters on the pathoanatomy and work-up. It then proceeds through the indications for, and literature behind, various treatment options. Finally, it ends with a treatment algorithm that can serve as an overall guide for clinicians. In each amenable chapter, we have included a "pearls and pitfalls" table that clearly delineates the key points that each author thinks are most important for their given topic. We hope the format of the book allows the reader to refer to it as a quick reference guide, but one that also offers an in-depth analysis of each topic through the text.

This book would not be possible without the contributions of the authors. They are all leaders in their fields, and each has extensive experience in treating patients with massive tears. They have generously donated their professional and personal time to contribute to this book. We are very grateful for their efforts, and we are honored to call them colleagues and friends.

The most instrumental person in the conception and production of this book is our Developmental Editor at Springer, Michael Griffin. He single-handedly pushed this process through to completion, even as timelines passed and attentions wandered. We are eternally indebted to him for his patience throughout the process, and his meticulous attention to details as drafts were revised. Thank you, Michael.

New York, NY, USA   Lawrence V. Gulotta, MD
                                                                    Edward V. Craig, MD, MPH

Contents

Contributors

Bashar Alolabi, MD, FRCSC Department of Orthopaedic Surgery, Sunnybrook Health Sciences Centre, Toronto, ON, Canada

Jeffrey D. Boatright, MD, MS Department of Orthopaedic Surgery, University of Virginia Medical Center, University of Virginia, Charlottesville, VA, USA

Stephen F. Brockmeier, MD Department of Orthopedic Surgery, University of Virginia, Charlottesville, VA, USA

Edward V. Craig, MD, MPH Professor of Cumor Surgery, Weill Cornell Medical School, New York, NY, USA

Attending Surgeon, Hospital for Special Surgery, New York, NY, USA

Austin J. Crow, MD Department of Orthopedic Surgery, University of Virginia, Charlottesville, VA, USA

Joshua S. Dines, MD Sports Medicine and Shoulder Service, Hospital for Special Surgery, New York, NY, USA

Department of Orthopaedic Surgery, Weill Cornell Medical College, New York, NY, USA

Seth C. Gamradt, MD Department of Orthopaedic Surgery, Keck School of Medicine of University of Southern California, Los Angeles, CA, USA

Brian Grawe, MD Sports Medicine and Shoulder Service, Hospital for Special Surgery, New York, NY, USA

Lawrence V. Gulotta, MD Sports Medicine and Shoulder Service, Hospital for Special Surgery, New York, NY, USA

Department of Orthopedic Surgery, Weill Cornell Medical School, New York, NY, USA

Anthony Ho, MD Department of Orthopaedic Surgery, George Washington University Hospital, Washington, DC, USA

Adam Z. Khan, BS Department of Orthopaedic Surgery, David Geffen School of Medicine at UCLA, Los Angeles, CA, USA

Gabrielle P. Konin, MD Department of Radiology and Imaging, Hospital for Special Surgery, New York, NY, USA

Department of Radiology and Imaging, Weill Cornell Medical College, New York, NY, USA

Moira M. McCarthy, MD Sports Medicine and Shoulder Surgery, Hospital for Special Surgery, New York, NY, USA

Jaydev B. Mistry, BA Rutgers New Jersey Medical School, Newark, NJ, USA

Andrew S. Neviaser, MD Department of Orthopaedic Surgery, George Washington University Hospital, Washington, DC, USA

Frank A. Petrigliano, MD Department of Orthopaedic Surgery, UCLA David Geffen School of Medicine, Los Angeles, CA, USA

Eric T. Ricchetti, MD Department of Orthopaedic Surgery, The Cleveland Clinic, Cleveland, OH, USA

Trevor P. Scott, MD Department of Orthopedic Surgery, UCLA Santa Monica Orthopaedic Center, Santa Monica, CA, USA

Russell F. Warren, MD Department of Orthopaedics, Hospital for Special Surgery, New York, NY, USA

Phillip N. Williams, MD Department of Orthopaedic Surgery, Hospital for Special Surgery, New York, NY, USA

Trevor P. Scott, Adam Z. Khan, and Frank A. Petrigliano

Pearls and Pitfalls

Pearls
- Acute cuff tears are often amenable to repair, even if they are massive.
- The degeneration-microtrauma theory is most accepted conceptualization of cuff disease.
- The rotator cuff is the major stabilizer of the shoulder during normal ROM. Small tears do not affect this capability, but larger tears may.
- Investigation and further understanding of these fundamental mechanisms will not only lead to better diagnostic and prognostic capabilities but will also aid in the development of better treatment modalities and adjunctive therapies for massive rotator cuff tears.PitfallsMuscle atrophy and fatty degeneration are associated with high failure rates in massive rotator cuff repairs.
- The exact pathway of muscle degeneration and fatty atrophy is not known and remains an area of active research.
- The pain generator in the setting of rotator cuff tears is not yet known, and research is ongoing.
- The exact size of cuff tear which leads to loss of force coupling and normal shoulder biomechanics is not yet known.

T.P. Scott, MD
Department of Orthopedic Surgery, UCLA Santa Monica Orthopaedic Center, 1250 16th Street, Santa Monica, CA 90404, USA
e-mail: tscott@mednet.ucla.edu

A.Z. Khan, BS
Department of Orthopaedic Surgery, David Geffen School of Medicine at UCLA, 10833 Le Conte Avenue, Los Angeles, CA 90095, USA
e-mail: Akhan881@gmail.com

F.A. Petrigliano, MD (✉)
UCLA David Geffen School of Medicine, 10833 Le Conte Avenue, 76-143-CHS, Los Angeles, CA 90095, USA
e-mail: fpetrigliano@gmail.com

Introduction

Rotator cuff injury is a common cause of shoulder pain accounting for 4.5 million clinic visits annually in the United States [1]. Massive tears account for between 10 and 40 % of all tears [2]. There is currently no consensus on the definition of a massive rotator cuff tear. Among the more commonly used definitions is that of Cofield et al. who described a massive rotator cuff tear as a tear with a diameter greater than 5 cm [3]. Another widely used definition is that used by

Gerber et al. that a massive rotator cuff tear is complete detachment of two or more cuff tendons from the proximal humerus [4]. Burkhart also suggested that massive tears be defined as tears greater than 5 cm and then further classified by pattern and edge mobility [5]. Posterosuperior tears are much more common than anterosuperior tears that extend down to the [6–10].

Massive tears may be amenable to surgery, especially when they are acute and tissue compliance is well maintained, but unfortunately, cases such as this are in the minority. Adhesions, scarring, fibrosis, tendon retraction, and poor tendon quality may all conspire to create a technically challenging repair [4, 11]. Furthermore, multiple studies have shown the re-tear rates following the repair of massive rotator cuff tears to be much greater than for smaller cuff tears. The purpose of this chapter is to review the pathophysiology and biomechanical changes that occur in the setting of massive rotator cuff tears and to discuss the clinical relevance of these functional alterations [12–18].

Historical Overview

The first documented description of tears of the tendons about the shoulder was reported by J.G. Smith in the *London Medical Gazette* in 1834 [12]. The connection between shoulder pain and the subacromial bursa was identified by Jaravay, and for several years this was believed to be the primary source of posttraumatic shoulder pain and stiffness, which was called "periarthritis humoscapularis" [13]. However, it was not until 1934 that Codman published his monograph on the anatomy of the rotator cuff and in which he discussed rotator cuff tears [19]. He was likely the first to identify that tears in the supraspinatus accounted for both difficulty with humeral abduction and shoulder pain. He was a proponent of early operative treatment and may have performed the first cuff repair in 1909 [20]. After Codman, McLaughlin and several other prominent surgeons including Armstrong, Smith-Peterson, Moseley, and Watson-Jones spent the next several decades publishing on the etiology and management of rotator cuff tears and there was emerging recognition that acromial abrasion might be a cause of rotator cuff injury [14–18].

Etiology

The etiology of rotator cuff tendinopathy and tears is commonly divided into extrinsic and intrinsic factors. Extrinsic factors are generally understood to mean compression or friction on the cuff by other shoulder structures. As early as 1924, Meyer described what would later come to be known as extrinsic factors when he discussed his "attrition theory" of musculotendinous rupture in the shoulder. He believed that many injuries which today would be described as rotator cuff tears could be attributed to chronic normal daily wear secondary to friction, and he believed supraspinatus tears originated superficially [21]. The concept of impingement was discussed in detail and classified by Neer in 1972. He identified spurs on the underside anterior 1/3 of the acromion, and he attributed degenerative changes of the acromion to friction from the cuff and humeral head. He associated tears of the cuff as being secondary to those same impinging forces. He described three stages to tears. Stage 1 was edema and hemorrhage in patients under 25, stage 2 was fibrosis and tendonitis in the 24–40 age group, and stage 3 were tendon ruptures and bone spurs in patients over 40 [22, 23]. Neer noted good results for focal acromioplasty of the anterior 1/3 of the lateral acromion. He also was much more aggressive with immediate surgical treatment with large complete tears than smaller injuries, correctly surmising that tendon retraction would make nonoperative treatment less successful and late surgical treatment challenging. For incomplete tears, he recommended an extended 9-month trial of nonoperative treatment, and for isolated complete supraspinatus tears, he performed surgery after a 6-week trial of nonoperative treatment [23].

Neer's hypothesis that impingement caused extrinsic cuff degeneration was further explored by Bigliani who identified three acromial shapes—flat, curved, and hooked—and noted that full-thickness rotator cuff tears were associated with hooked acromial shape [24]. It also was recognized that impingement could occur against multiple surfaces, given the remarkable range of motion of the glenohumeral joint. Thus, it could be due not only to acromial shape but also to arthritic changes of the acromioclavicular (AC) joint or the coracoacromial ligament [25]. Further compression of the cuff, biceps tendon, and/or subacromial bursa between the humeral head and the acromion, AC joint, or coracoacromial ligament all may be related to motion of the humeral head [25, 26]. Also, the relatively shallow glenohumeral joint puts the joint at risk for instability that can lead to increased humeral head translation. Translation, in turn, can initiate or exacerbate impingement [25, 27].

Many authors have suggested that if impingement on superior structures actually leads to tears, then the majority of tears should be on the bursal side of the cuff. Yet, multiple studies have suggested that the majority of cuff tears start on the articular surface [28, 29]. Those authors have suggested that arthritic AC changes, and morphologic changes of the acromion and the CA ligament, which were thought to cause cuff impingement via extrinsic compression, may in fact simply be correlated with age. It is also possible the impingement changes may actually be a secondary response to intrinsic tendon changes [28, 30, 31]. Moreover, studies by Neer and others have shown that many patients with tears never performed hard labor or vigorous overhead activity [22].

This, however, does not discount impingement as a major factor in cuff tears; intrinsic factors suggest that the cuff fails on the articular side because there is more fibrocartilage, which has a lower tensile strength, on the articular side which is the side that may also undergo more strain [29, 32]. These findings have helped give rise to the theory that it is actually internal impingement of the cuff on the humeral head which results in tears [33]. In all likelihood, degenerative cuff tears are secondary to extrinsic compression combined with intrinsic factors. A recent rat study showed the rats whose cuffs were subject to both compression and overuse, as opposed to one or the other alone, had much greater rates of tendinopathy [34].

The degeneration-microtrauma theory [35] is the most widely accepted conceptualization of the events resulting in the development of rotator cuff disease. It describes *intrinsic degeneration* of the rotator cuff tendon secondary to age-related changes such as changes in collagen-type

synthesis, vascular changes, hypoxia, or oxidative stress. This degeneration makes the tendon more susceptible to damage; repetitive stresses cause micro-injuries— i.e., reduction in the number of functional fibers in the tendon puts increasing load on the remaining fibers—which are not given enough time to heal before further trauma occurs. It should be noted that most studies, which aim to elucidate the pathophysiology of rotator cuff degeneration and rupture, are in animal models, and it is important to recognize the anatomic, biologic, and functional limitations inherent to animal research model systems.

Pathophysiology

Degeneration of the rotator cuff tendon results from a variety of intrinsic factors including but not limited to age-related degeneration, inflammation, vascular changes, and oxidative stress. Among these elements, the key factor leading to rotator cuff weakness and degeneration is aging.

Epidemiologic studies indicate a positive correlation between patient age and rotator cuff tear incidence. An ultrasound study performed by Tempelhof and colleagues [36] screened more than 400 asymptomatic volunteers and found an increase in tear prevalence with increasing age. Cuff tear incidence increased from 13 % in the 50–59-year-old age group to 51 % in the 80–89-year-old age group. The high incidence of asymptomatic rotator cuff tears in the aging population brings about the question of whether rotator cuff degeneration is in fact a pathologic process or could be considered a part of the "normal" aging process. Furthermore, the clinically relevant question of how an asymptomatic cuff tear develops into a painful, function-limiting, symptomatic tear requires further investigation.

With increasing age, many histologic changes have been observed. A study by Hashimoto and colleagues [37] described 7 characteristic features of age-related degeneration (Fig. 1.1). Thinning and disorganization of collagen fibers, myxoid degeneration (connective tissue replaced by mucus), and hyaline degeneration were observed in all 80 patient samples in the study. Other degenerative changes observed were vascular proliferation

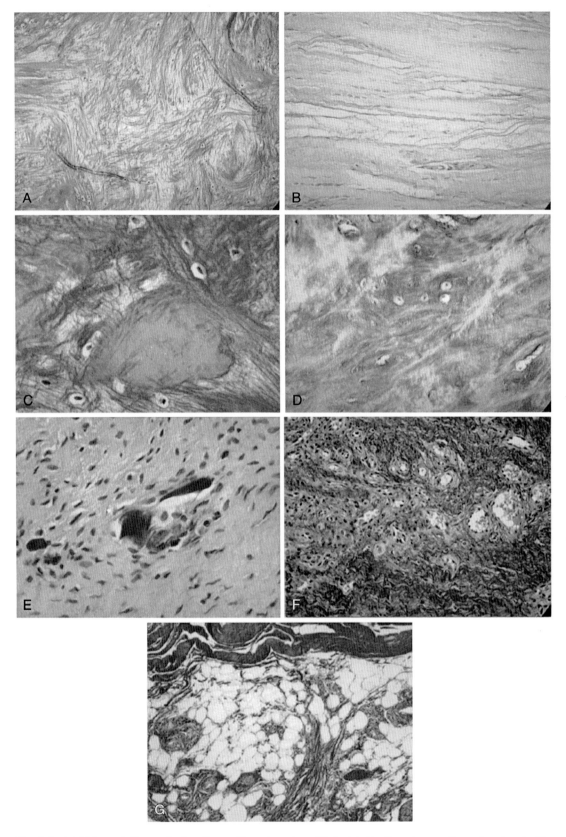

Fig. 1.1 (**a**) Thin and disorganized collagen fibers in the torn tendon (large tear, 10× magnification). (**b**) Split collagen fibers replaced with myxoid degeneration (large tear, 20×). (**c**) Hyaline degeneration; chondrocyte-like cells are visible near hyalines areas, (large tear, 20×). (**d**) Chondrocytes with lacunae, intracellular matrix

(34 %), fatty infiltration (33 %), chondroid metaplasia (21 %), and calcification (19 %).

Longo and colleagues [38] subsequently reevaluated the histology of rotator cuff tears. In the torn rotator cuff samples, they found increased waviness and disorganization (loss of parallel architecture) of collagen fibers and an increase in vascularity. Furthermore, rounding of tenocyte nuclei—normally flat and spindle shaped—to the point where they almost resembled chondrocytes was observed in the torn cuff samples.

In a rat model, overuse of the rotator cuff tendon led to downregulation of TGF-β1. Another study by Perry and colleagues [39] looked at rat model of repetitive microtrauma and found acute increases (peak at 3 days) in VEGF and subacute (8 weeks) increases in inducible cyclooxygenase (COX-2). The results of these studies not only support the repetitive microtrauma theory, but they imply the presence of acute inflammation as well as a central role for angiogenic mediators.

Oxidative stress and the production of reactive oxygen species (ROS) are implicated in the degeneration and pathologic destruction of a variety of different tissue types. One of the main mechanisms by which ROS are thought to contribute to tissue degeneration is through the activation of the intrinsic apoptotic pathway. Studies by Yuan and colleagues [40] exhibited an increase in apoptotic cells at the cuff tear edge (34 %) as compared with control (13 %). In addition to induction of apoptosis, oxidative stress has been shown to induce cuff degeneration through induction of two other auxiliary factors: c-Jun N-terminal protein kinase (JNK), a mitogen-induced protein kinase (MAPK) expressed intracellularly, and matrix metalloproteinase-1 (MMP-1), an enzyme present in the extracellular environment. In vivo, JNK and MMP-1 expression were increased in torn supraspinatus tendon specimens as well as in tendon specimens that were exposed to the ROS peroxide [41] (Fig. 1.2).

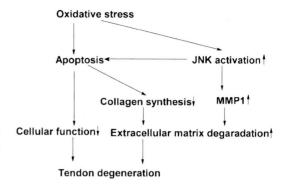

Fig. 1.2 Model of potential pathway of oxidative stress and apoptosis in rotator cuff degeneration (Wang et al. [41])

MMPs are responsible for maintaining the dynamic homeostasis of the extracellular matrix (ECM). They are in a delicate equilibrium with endogenous inhibitors of their activity: tissue inhibitors of MMPs (TIMPs) [42]. A disruption of balance in the expression and activity of MMP and TIMP is associated with pathologic change in overuse tendinopathies [43] as well as specifically rotator cuff tears [44]. MMP-1 is found to be in low concentration in normal tendon and increased in damaged supraspinatus tendon [45, 46], along with MMP-9 and MMP-13 [46]. MMPs and JNK secondary to oxidative stress are believed to contribute to the loss of tissue architecture and weakened structure in the rotator cuff.

Early histologic studies of injured rotator cuff showed little to no evidence of chronic inflammation [37, 47, 48]. Some studies have been able to show the expression of inflammatory cytokines and mediators [49–52], but many histologic studies are unable to demonstrate the presence of actual inflammatory cells [37, 47, 53–55]. A limitation to these studies is that samples were obtained in the later stages of rotator cuff tear progression. However, more recent data published by Millar and colleagues [56] demonstrated the first in vivo human evidence of an inflammatory infiltrate in early tendinopathy.

Fig. 1.1 (continued) stained with alcian blue (large tear 20×). (**e**) Calcific deposits in tendon between spindle-shaped fibroblasts and collagen fibers (massive tear, 40×). (**f**) Proliferation of small vessels in all tendon layers and edema (articular surface tear, 20×). (**g**) Fatty infiltration in the proximal tendon, distributed from middle to deep tissue layer (large tear, 10×). **a**, **c**, **f**, and **g** are stained with Masson trichrome; **b** and **e** are stained with hematoxylin and eosin; **d** is stained with alcian blue (Hashimoto et al. [37])

They found the subscapular tendons of patients with supraspinatus tears had an increased number of macrophages, mast cells, and T cells as well as a higher vessel density compared with the torn supraspinatus and control subscapularis tissue.

There exists some controversy with regard to the role that vascular changes play in the degeneration of the rotator cuff tendon. The traditional line of belief is that a "critical" zone of hypovascular tissue exists 10–15 mm from the insertion of the supraspinatus tendon, which makes this area more prone to tears [19, 57, 58]. Furthermore, via ultrasonography imaging, it is a well-documented phenomenon that blood supply to the rotator cuff decreases with age, especially past the age of 40 [59].

Yet, histologic data is more equivocal in regard to the significance of this hypovascular zone to cuff pathology. In the majority of histologic studies, hypervascular tissue is observed around the cuff tear site—a response to injury believed to proliferate from the subsynovial layer long after the original injury [37, 55]. Rathbun and colleagues [60] found that reduced perfusion to the rotator cuff is observed only when the arm is fully adducted. However, a histologic study by Brooks and colleagues [61] found a decrease in the degree of filling, size, and number of vessels in the proximal 15 mm to the supraspinatus insertion. Interestingly, they found this same pattern in the infraspinatus, which tears much less frequently.

Despite equivocal histologic and imaging data on the vascular changes that may occur during the development of rotator cuff pathology, there is some molecular data being uncovered that supports a role for local hypoxia in the development of rotator cuff pathology. Benson and colleagues [62] observed within the torn supraspinatus an increase in expression of BNip3, a proapoptotic cytokine of the BcL-2 family, as well as hypoxia-inducible factor-1α, indicating a connection between local hypoxia and inflammation-induced apoptosis. Furthermore, Millar and colleagues [50] showed that hypoxia, in addition to inducing apoptotic mediators, will induce a change in collagen synthesis—decreasing collagen I synthesis and increasing collagen III synthesis, as well as increasing key inflammatory mediators: monocyte chemotactic protein (MCP)-1, interleukin (IL)-6, and IL-8. Additionally, as will be discussed in a later section, local hypoxia may drive the differentiation of pluripotent cells to an adipocyte lineage.

A retrospective ultrasonographic study of patients evaluated for shoulder pain performed by Baumgarten and colleagues [63] found that a history of smoking is correlated with an increased risk of rotator cuff tears; they also observed a time-dependent and dose-dependent relationship between smoking and rotator cuff tear incidence. This observation may be due to microvascular disease; however, a causal relationship has not been well established.

Abboud and colleagues [64] found that increased total cholesterol, LDL, and triglycerides were all present in patients with rotator cuff pathology compared with controls. They also found lower HDL levels in patients with rotator cuff disease compared with control patients. Whether elevated cholesterol is actually an independent predictor of cuff pathology or simply an ancillary factor that accompanies advanced age is unclear.

Various studies have indicated that genetics may be involved in the pathogenesis of rotator cuff tears [65–68]. Although no specific gene mutations or abnormalities have been correlated with rotator cuff tear incidence, there is an epidemiologic data indicating a genetic component to rotator cuff disease. Harvie and colleagues [69] showed that siblings have a 2.42 relative risk of developing full-thickness tears compared with controls.

An interesting alternative theory compares rotator cuff degeneration to CNS damage. In the CNS, repeated stimulation and release of glutamate results in "excitotoxicity" and leads to apoptosis of neurons [70]. The neural theory of tendinopathy [71] follows a similar line of thinking: neural overstimulation, secondary to tendon overuse, results in recruitment of inflammatory cells and apoptosis. Hart and colleagues [72] have already documented this inflammatory cell recruitment, secondary to neural overstimulation, in vivo. The key molecules implicated driving degeneration are glutamate and substance P.

There is some evidence showing substance P overexpression association with rotator cuff pathology [73]. Furthermore, Molloy and colleagues [70] found an increase in various glutamate-signaling proteins in rat supraspinatus tendon following overuse. Further evidence in support of this theory is limited.

The development of symptoms related to rotator cuff pathology is poorly understood. Having an asymptomatic rotator cuff tear increases the risk of future symptomatic progression [74]. Yet many asymptomatic tears do not develop into symptomatic tears. There is also data correlating increasing tear size with symptomatic presentation; Yamaguchi and colleagues performed an ultrasonographic study of 588 patients and found that in patients with bilateral tears, the symptomatic tear was larger than the asymptomatic tear and in symptomatic shoulders the average cuff tear size is 30 % greater than in asymptomatic shoulders [75].

Definitive histologic evidence of inflammation within a degenerating rotator cuff is elusive, but many proinflammatory cytokines and inflammatory mediators such as COX-2, leukotriene B4, and PGE_2 are overexpressed in rotator cuff injuries. It is hypothesized the painful symptoms of rotator cuff disease could be mediated by COX-2 and PGE_2 [35, 76]. There is still limited data in support of these theories, and further investigation needs to be performed.

Muscle Degeneration

In orthopedic literature, the phenomenon of adipocyte accumulation in and around skeletal muscle is referred to by a variety of names: fatty infiltration, fatty degeneration, or fatty change. A histologic study, by Meyer and colleagues [77], showed normal-appearing muscle fibers with adipocyte infiltration, but no degeneration—suggesting fatty infiltration as the appropriate terminology. Itoigawa and colleagues [78], however, believe the "infiltrating" adipocytes to actually be differentiating from muscle stem cells and therefore believed fatty degeneration to be accurate. As this debate is ongoing, this chapter will use these terms interchangeably.

Muscle atrophy is commonly seen with disuse and the unloading of tensile force on the skeletal muscle. Yet, the rotator cuff is unique in that when injured, a fatty-fibrous degeneration, in addition to disuse atrophy, is observed. It is currently unclear if fatty degeneration of the rotator cuff is suggestive of a failed repair mechanism that predisposes to tears or if it is simply intrinsic to the normal degenerative process [79].

The tear of the rotator cuff tendon, detachment from the bone, and subsequent unloading of stress on the rotator cuff tendon and muscle lead to changes in the muscle and tendon structure. Structural changes include myofibril disorganization—decreased sarcomere length and number—followed by a reduction in muscle mass and volume rather than fiber death [80]. This disuse atrophy, resulting from an extended period of muscle retraction, leads to a pattern of progressive fibrosis and increased fat content that accumulated at intrafascicular, extrafascicular, and intratendinous sites within the muscle [77, 81, 82]. Fatty infiltration and muscle atrophy are seen throughout the tendon and muscle [79]. The degree of fatty infiltration and muscle atrophy progression in rotator cuff tears is positively correlated with patient age, tear size (length and width), location, full-thickness involvement [83], and chronicity [81] of the tear. Suprascapular neuropathy or denervation secondary to muscle retraction and resulting neuropraxia has also been implicated in contributing to the degree of these pathologic changes [84–89].

Muscle atrophy and fatty degeneration are progressive and often irreversible adverse histologic changes that occur throughout the tendon and muscle [82, 90, 91]. While surgical repair may prevent further progression of muscle atrophy and fatty degeneration, it often does not reverse established preoperative fatty degeneration and atrophy [90–94]. Many of the histologic changes noted in rotator cuff tendon are also reflected in the rotator cuff muscle. The ECM is extensively reorganized and remodeled by the same family of matrix metalloproteinases (MMPs) during the progression of muscle atrophy following a rotator cuff tear. MMP-2,

MMP-9, and MMP-13 overexpression has been associated with muscle atrophy [82, 90, 91]. It has also been hypothesized that the Akt-mammalian target of rapamycin (mTOR) pathway is central to the development of muscle atrophy [95]. Increased mTOR and Akt activity is associated with an inhibition of nuclear factor kappa B (NF-κB) and forkhead transcription factor (FOXO). Both NF-κB and FOXO regulate increased expression of proteins associated with muscle atrophy [96, 97]. In chronic human supraspinatus tears, these proteinases along with NF-κB were upregulated [98] (Fig. 1.3).

The exact source of the adipocytes that contribute to fatty degeneration of the rotator cuff is still not certain. The current hypotheses are (1) preexisting adipocytes are stimulated and proliferate within the muscle, (2) resident pluripotent stem cells are signaled to differentiate into mature adipocytes, and (3) adipocytes are recruited from extramuscular sources [78]. Of the three, the current molecular research indicates that the differentiation of local stem cells, known as mesenchymal stem cells (MSCs), appears to be the most likely source of adipocytes during fatty degeneration. Transcription factors of the MRF family implicated in the differentiation of myoblasts into mature myocytes are MYoD, Myf-5, myogenin, and MRF4 [100, 101]. Furthermore, two different families of transcription factors are believed to differentiate pre-adipocytes into mature adipocytes; these are CCAT/enhancer-binding proteins (C/EBPs) and peroxisome proliferator-activated receptors (PPARs) [78, 102, 103]. In an ovine model of rotator cuff tear, real-time PCR analysis identified increases in Myf-5 and PPARγ expression after tenotomy and subsequent increases in Myf-5 and C/EBPβ expression post repair [104]. Furthermore, the Wnt signaling pathway has also been identified to be central to adipogenesis of MSCs [78, 105–107]. More specifically, in vitro culture of a murine myogenic cell line (C2C12) in an adipogenic culture media resulted in diminished Wnt10b expression and increased expression of PPARγ and C/EBPα; this expression pattern was subsequently confirmed in vivo by gene expression analysis in a rotator cuff tear rat model [78].

Fatty degeneration predominates in the distal portion of the rotator cuff muscle near the musculotendinous junction [78, 88, 91, 108]; at this region of the cuff, there also exists a more sustained decrease in Wnt10b as well as an increase in PPARγ and C/EBPα [78]. Two mechanisms are implicated in driving these changes in protein signaling. The first is muscle retraction: mechanical stretching of muscle tissue was shown to increase Wnt10 signaling and inhibit adipogenesis [109]. Therefore, retraction of muscle tissue is thought to have the opposite effect on Wnt signaling and thus promotes adipocyte proliferation. The second mechanism is that local hypoxia can contribute to adipocyte proliferation through trans-differentiation of myoblasts [106]. This trans-differentiation is associated with increased PPARγ expression, which is also observed during hypoxic conditions [106]. Furthermore, two different studies have found increased expression of hypoxia-inducible factor 1 and VEGF to be associated with the development of fatty infiltration [62, 110].

Rotator Cuff Healing at the Bone-Tendon Junction

The normal insertion of tendon into the bone is comprised of four distinct zones: tendon, unmineralized fibrocartilage, mineralized fibrocartilage, and bone [111]. Following rotator cuff repair, the tendon-to-bone interface does not recapitulate the native enthesis but rather forms a reactive scar [112, 113].

One suggestion is that healing is affected by the vascular supply to the rotator cuff [114]. As described in the aforementioned histologic studies [37, 38], vascular proliferation is often noted in torn rotator cuff muscle. In contrast, Gamradt and colleagues [115] have found that the healing cuff tendon is fairly avascular and that a significant amount of the vascular supply to the healing cuff originates from the bone [46, 116].

Other than decreased vascular supply, it is also believed that poor cuff healing is a result of disorganized temporal expression of cytokines. Furthermore, slow and incomplete bony ingrowth

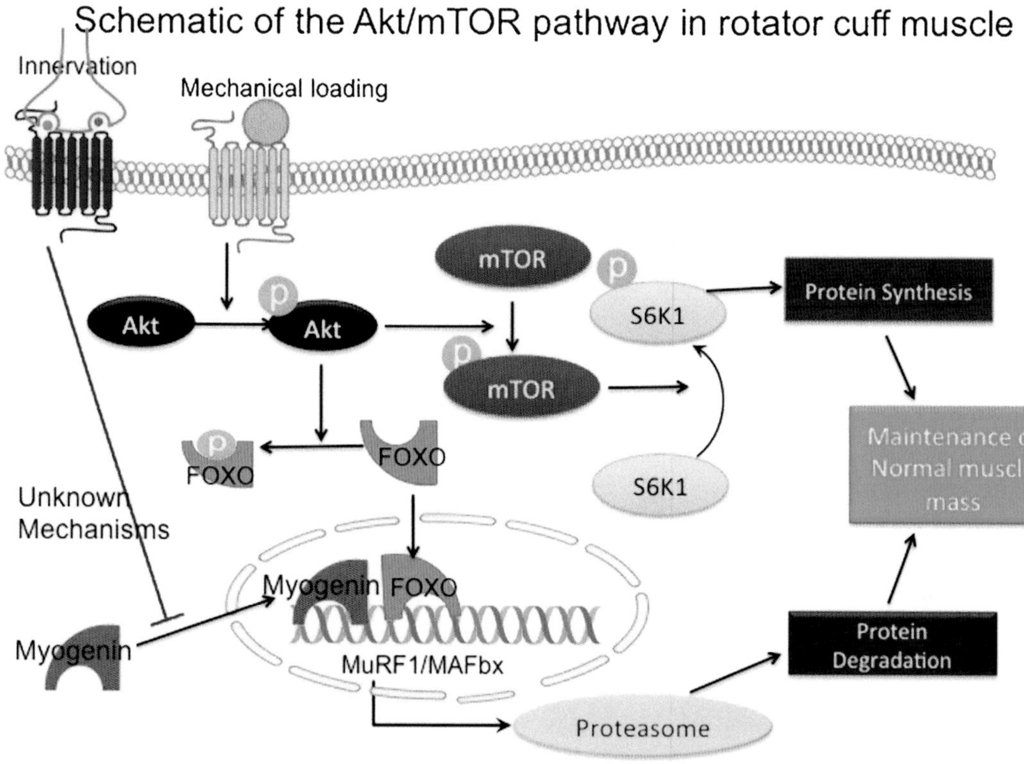

Fig. 1.3 Akt/mTOR signaling pathway in the rotator cuff muscle. A balance between protein degradation and synthesis maintains muscle mass. Akt-mTOR-S6K1 pathway stimulates protein synthesis secondary to normal mechanical loading of muscle tissue. Via an undetermined mechanism, normal muscle innervation inhibits MuRF-1/MAFbx overexpression through myogenin activation (Liu et al. [99])

into the tendon from the prepared tuberosity, inflammatory cells that precipitate scar formation at tendon-bone interface, and a scarce population of undifferentiated stem cells at the bone-tendon interface all may prevent proper healing [112].

Three stages are involved in the degeneration and healing of the rotator cuff: (1) inflammatory phase, (2) repair phase, and (3) remodeling phase [117]. Various cytokines are expressed throughout different time points within these three stages to facilitate proper tendon-to-bone healing. During the inflammatory phase, the fibrovascular scar tissue is produced in the rotator cuff following an infiltrate of mast cells and macrophages [56]. These macrophages will secrete signaling molecule such as transforming growth factor β1 (TGF-β1): a cytokine known to increase collagen formation and proteinase activity [118]. After the inflammatory phase, fibroblasts are activated within the repair phase. These activated fibroblasts express a variety of cytokines, which are described below.

PDGF-β is believed to play a central role in the repair of tendons and ligaments. It has been shown to promote chemotaxis, extracellular matrix production, surface integrin expression, cell proliferation, and revascularization in fibroblasts [119–122]. Improved mechanical properties stem from PDGF-β stimulating increased collagen I production. In an ovine model of rotator cuff repair, sheep treated with PDGF-β had improved histologic scores and load-to-failure rates [123]. The TGF-β family of proteins is integral to normal fetal development, modulation of scar tissue after a wound, and tendon-to-bone healing [112]. Varied expression levels of two different TGF-β isoforms modulate the amount of scar that forms at the tendon-bone healing site

[124, 125]. Treatment of the healing enthesis with TGF-β3 produces a more favorable collagen I to collagen III ratio to withstand increased tensile strength [126]. The BMP family, which is a subset of the TGF-β superfamily, also plays a role in healing of the enthesis via bony ingrowth. BMP-12, BMP-13, and BMP-14 are three cytokines [127], which contribute to the synthesis of fibrocartilage, induction of neotendon, and ligament formation. During the initial inflammatory phase of tendon healing, IGF-1 is activated. It contributes to chemotaxis as well as proliferation of fibroblasts and inflammatory cells to the site of injury [112]. In vivo, it increases cellular proliferation, enhances matrix synthesis, improves tendon mechanical properties, and reduces time to functional recovery [128–130]. FGF-1 and bFGF (also known as FGF-2) are both central modulators of angiogenesis and mesenchymal cell mitogenesis [112]. The more potent mitogen is bFGF, and during healing it helps initiate the formation of granulation tissue [131–133] and induction of fibroblast collagenase with a dose-dependent increase in type III collagen expression levels [134, 135]. Furthermore, bFGF expression by fibroblasts is also associated with improved tendon healing [134–137], cell proliferation, cell migration, collagen production, and angiogenesis [138–141]. Increased vascular supply is also central to proper rotator cuff healing. Vascular endothelial growth factor (VEGF) contributes to neovascularization and, in several models, has been observed at the site of the healing enthesis [142–145].

Just as rotator cuff pathology is a degenerative process resulting from a variety of influences, proper rotator cuff healing is also a multifactorial process. Therefore, rotator cuff repairs often fail through a combination of barriers to proper healing, which can be characterized into three broad categories: biologic factors, technical errors, and traumatic failure [114], of which the biologic factors may be the most pertinent. The biologic factors that underlie improper rotator cuff healing are the patient age, level of fatty degeneration, amount of muscle atrophy, cuff vascularity, and tear size. Furthermore, medical comorbidities such as diabetes, nicotine use, and NSAID use have also been found to be detrimental in rotator cuff healing.

Fatty degeneration and muscle atrophy are both independent predictors of poor functional outcomes following rotator cuff repair [90]. Increases in fatty infiltration and muscle atrophy can increase the tension applied to the repair site as these degenerative changes decrease the compliance of the musculotendinous unit. This phenomenon has been confirmed in both animal models and clinical studies [146]. Postoperative radiographic assessment demonstrates higher re-tear rates to be associated with an increased degree of fatty degeneration and muscle atrophy [90, 147, 148]. Although degenerative changes in the rotator cuff muscle are often irreversible [82, 90, 91], the further progression of these changes can be diminished by surgical repair [90–94]. Therefore, earlier repair can lead to greater recovery of muscle and tendon elasticity [149], lower re-tear rates, and improved clinical results [150].

As mentioned earlier, there is a positive correlation between patient age and cuff tear incidence. Several studies have found that increasing patient age is also correlated with decreased healing rates postoperatively [151–157]. One contributing factor could be insufficient postoperative vascular supply in elderly patients. Contrast-enhanced ultrasound suggests that blood supply to the tendon has an effect on healing [59, 114, 115], and diminished blood supply to the rotator cuff is observed with increasing age, especially in patients over 40 [59].

There are multiple factors intrinsic to the cuff tear itself that can also contribute to poor outcomes following repair. These include the number of cuff tendons torn [154], the quality of the cuff tendon, as well as the initial tear size [152, 154–157]. A study by Nho and colleagues [157] established that with each centimeter increase in tear size, there is a twofold increase in risk of persistent tear or re-tear following repair. Finally, postoperative NSAID (indomethacin and celecoxib) administration in a rat model has been demonstrated to effect tendon-to-bone healing. Animals treated with NSAIDs showed decreased collagen organization and maturation as well as a decreased load-to-failure ratio at 4- and 8-week time points following rotator cuff repair [158]. However, there have been no clinical studies to confirm the detrimental effects of NSAID use on rotator cuff healing.

Biomechanics of Rotator Cuff Tear

The effect of a massive rotator cuff tear on the biomechanics of the shoulder can only be understood in the context of normal shoulder biomechanics. The purpose of the shoulder is to position the hand in space, and the glenohumeral joint has the greatest range of motion of any joint to accomplish this function. The design of the shoulder provides a balance between motion, force transmission, and stability: the rotator cuff contributes to all three.

Shoulder motion is complex, but a reasonable understanding of it can be gained by considering the shoulder through the lens of planar and 3D motion. Planar motion consists of spinning, sliding, and rolling. Spinning is essentially rotation of the humeral head on the fixed glenoid; the instantaneous center of rotation is at the center of the humeral head. Sliding is translation of the humerus on the glenoid, and the instantaneous center of the rotation is at the center of glenoid curvature. Finally rolling is a motion between moving and fixed segments where the contact points are constantly changing [159]. The shoulder is essentially a spherical spinning joint with a small amount of translation [160] (Fig. 1.4). Alternately shoulder motion can be thought of in terms of Eulerian angles as along the x axis (along the humeral shaft), y axis (lateral to the scapular plane), and the z axis (perpendicular to the scapula). Shoulder motion can be described by angular motion in those planes and is known to be sequence dependent [159, 161] (Fig. 1.5).

The exact contribution of each aspect of the cuff to shoulder motion remains a subject of great debate. In general, however, what is known is that the supraspinatus assists the deltoid in some capacity to elevate the humerus, and it also externally rotates the arm [162–166]. Whether this is primarily after the first 30° of abduction as

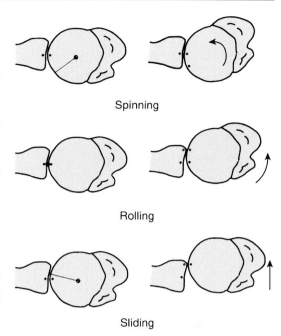

Spinning

Rolling

Sliding

Fig. 1.4 The three planar types of motion (spinning, rolling, and sliding) all occur in the glenohumeral joint (Itoi et al. [161])

postulated remains undetermined, many authors have argued that in fact the supraspinatus is likely most important in the first 30° of abduction as that is where its mechanical advantage is greatest [162, 164, 167]. The subscapularis internally rotates the humerus, and the infraspinatus and teres minor externally rotate the humerus [166]. The subscapularis, infraspinatus, and teres minor also may elevate or depress the humerus depending on the position of the humerus. The inferior cuff likely contributes to some aspect of abduction though this is probably as a stabilizer [164, 168].

The rotator cuff also provides a significant contribution to the stability of the glenohumeral joint. Stability of the glenohumeral joint is provided by a combination of static and dynamic stabilizers. The static stabilizers primarily contribute to stability at the extremes of joint motion and consist of both soft tissue and bony components; but they are mostly independent of the cuff. The glenoid itself provides some stability via approximately 25–30 % contact with humeral head, which is increased to 33 % by an intact labrum.

1–3'–1" ROTATION SEQUENCE
[LEFT SHOULDER (PA VIEW)]

A
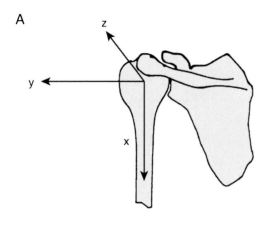

B
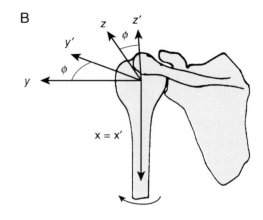

C
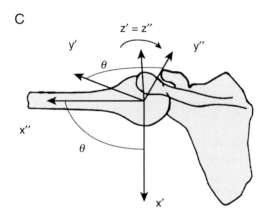

D
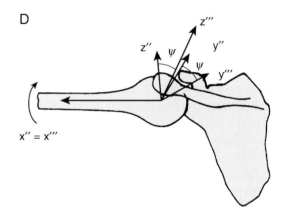

Fig. 1.5 Glenohumeral motion in three dimensions as described by the Eulerian system. (**a**) Neutral position, (**b**) First rotation ϕ: axial rotation about x axis represents the plane of elevation, (**c**) Second rotation θ: rotation about z' axis represents arm elevation, (**d**) Third rotation ψ: axial rotation about x'' axis represents humeral rotation (Itoi et al. [161])

The glenohumeral articulation, even when the labrum is included, is shallow and relatively unstable, but stability at the extremes of motion is greatly increased by the ligamentocapsular structures. The coracoacromial ligament is a key superior stabilizer of the shoulder; the superior glenohumeral ligament prevents inferior subluxation; the middle glenohumeral ligament blends with the subscapular tendon and provides anterior stability especially in mid-abduction and external rotation; the inferior glenohumeral ligament functions as a primary anterior-posterior stabilizer in abduction. The inferior glenohumeral ligament's anterior band contributes stability in flexion or external rotation, whereas its posterior band is the key ligamentous stabilizer in extension [169]. Finally negative intra-articular pressure prevents subluxation, especially inferiorly [170, 171].

While these structures are important to stability of the shoulder, especially at the extremes of motion, the cuff is an important component of dynamic shoulder stabilization. In fact, it is probably the major stabilizer in normal shoulder range of motion. All muscles of the shoulder, especially the rotator cuff, provide passive resistance to humeral displacement, which is demonstrated by the fact that muscle removal but not cuff paralysis significantly increased the range of motion of the joint [164, 172]. The muscles of the rotator cuff also provide stability through a barrier effect. The anterior barrier to subluxation is provided by subscapularis, and superiorly the supraspinatus provides a spacer between the head and acromion [173, 174].

Most important, though, is contraction of the cuff musculature, which is probably essential in creating joint compression via the "compression-contracture" model of stability. The contraction of the cuff musculature both centers the head and compresses the head against the glenoid concavity which in turn prevents lateral translation [42, 164]. The balanced compression of the anterior and posterior aspects of the cuff leads to the idea of force coupling first suggested in the work of Inman and later Saha [175, 176]. The long head of the biceps tendon, often abnormal in the setting of rotator cuff injury, may help compress the head and likely help compensate for the loss of stability with cuff injury [177]. Overall the muscles of the rotator cuff are key to glenohumeral stability and allow the other muscles of the shoulder to move the stabilized glenohumeral joint.

The final component of shoulder biomechanics that bears examination is the force generated by the muscles across the glenohumeral joint. Joint reaction forces are greatest at 90° of abduction, as are joint contact pressure, though only in the setting of an intact cuff creating normal force coupling [178, 179]. Massive cuff tears decrease this effect, but small isolated tears of the supraspinatus do not appear to have a major effect (Fig. 1.6) [178].

Multiple studies have attempted to determine the activity of the cuff muscles in various arm functions aside from generation of force coupling. Duchenne's earliest studies used galvanic measures, but more recent studies have primarily utilized EMG. The majority of studies have examined the relative importance of the supraspinatus and the deltoid to arm abduction. It remains subject to debate, but the supraspinatus is likely most essential at the generation of abduction, though if this is due more to stabilization as part of the cuff or due to its moment arm giving it a

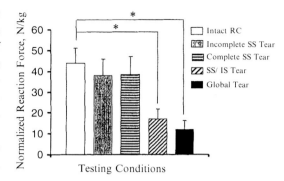

Fig. 1.6 The glenohumeral force normalized for the weight of the arm in each of the above testing conditions demonstrates a decrease in joint reaction force in large tears (Parsons et al. [178])

mechanical advantage is unclear. It also is likely a key centralizer of the humeral head due to the location of its moment arm [180]. Meanwhile the infraspinatus and teres minor work as humeral head depressors, but as noted above that is position dependent [164]. However, overall it seems that the cuff is most important for stabilization as in vivo EMG studies suggest that the cuff musculature is activated prior to other muscles in shoulder motion [181].

Pathological Effect of a Rotator Cuff Tear on Shoulder Biomechanics

The exact etiology of massive rotator cuff tears and their natural history remain undetermined. Most models suggest that the tears initiate in the anterior supraspinatus insertion and then spread posteriorly [25, 182]. Once initiated, a tear results in greater stress across the remaining fibers at the edge. When the force on the remaining fibers exceeds maximal tensile strength, this scenario can lead to propagation of the tear. The edges of the tear have compromised blood flow and are exposed to the lytic enzymes present in synovial fluid, both of which impede healing [20]. Once a tear has become large enough, activation of the deltoid may actually create a significant amount of shear stress that can damage the joint or even propagate the tear further [179]. This may also lead to further cuff degeneration as the remaining

Uncoupling of Essential Forces

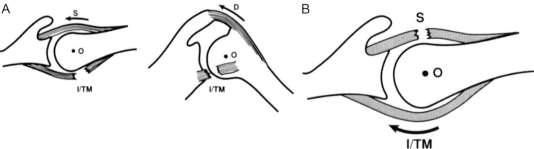

Fig. 1.7 Transverse plane force coupling is disrupted by massive tears of the posterior rotator cuff, including the infraspinatus and teres minor (**a**). Loss of force plane coupling transversely due to a tear of the subscapularis (**b**). *O* center of rotation, *S* subscapularis, *D* deltoid, *I* infraspinatus, *TM* teres minor (Burkhart et al. [186])

superior cuff may be compressed between the elevated humeral head and the acromion. Erosion of the superior glenoid rim may also hamper the remaining shoulder musculature's ability to stabilize the humeral head against the glenoid [174].

Massive Rotator Cuff Tears and Shoulder Biomechanics

Patients with rotator cuff tears, even massive tears, have a wide range of clinical symptoms; many are even asymptomatic (though they frequently develop symptoms over time) [183]. As a result, the exact function of the rotator cuff and the subsequent effect of cuff tears have remained a subject of great debate.

As discussed previously, the glenohumeral joint functions primarily as a spherical joint with a small amount of translation to allow that motion [184, 185]. Within that context, the cuff maintains concavity compression to stabilize the joint so that it may be moved by other shoulder girdle muscles; it also functions to steer and rotate the joint [164, 176, 181]. This data implies that the major function of the rotator cuff is to maintain dynamic stability of the glenohumeral joint, which in turn helps position the hand in space. Probably less importantly, the cuff also functions to move the joint [181].

Small tears isolated to the supraspinatus have a minimal effect on shoulder biomechanics in cadaver and computer models where pain is not a relevant issue. Massive tears, on the other hand, disrupt the stabilizing mechanism of the rotator cuff. However, if there is normal force coupling, then the shoulder can potentially function normally, even in the setting of a large tear. Burkhart and his coauthors suggested that if the subscapularis and posterior cuff engage in transverse force coupling in the transverse plane and the inferior cuff and deltoid are balanced coronally, then the humerus can rotate in a stable fashion [186] (Fig. 1.7). This led them to recommend partial repair without complete closure of massive tears if force coupling could be established. Moreover, a subsequent study indicated that an intact teres minor and subscapsularis were key to good function after surgery [186, 187]. As Burkhart and other authors have noted, patients can often tolerate a tear of the supraspinatus and superior half of the infraspinatus, but a tear of the inferior half of the infraspinatus may lead to a loss of balanced force coupling and functional impairment [5, 178, 188, 189]. If the tear becomes large enough that the force coupling is lost, then the deltoid becomes a destabilizing force that pulls the humeral head superiorly. A boutonniere deformity can develop where the inferior cuff actually becomes the humeral head elevator. This can also damage the superior glenoid and labrum, further destabilizing the glenohumeral joint [174].

Rotator cuff tears can also result in the loss of the barrier effect of the supraspinatus, and potentially other cuff muscles, which can also allow abnormal head kinematics, especially superior head migration. The loss of the barrier, in concert with destabilizing effect of the deltoid, may be what causes massive cuff tears to progress to cuff tear arthropathy [174]. The effect of tears on the joint reaction forces remains unclear. Parsons et al. found that joint reactive force was decreased in complete tears of the supraspinatus; but Hansen found the joint-reactive force to be increased at early abduction. If joint reactive force is decreased, it could indicate at least partial loss of the stabilizing contraction compression mechanism [160, 178].

The question of when a large tear begins to alter the biomechanics of the shoulder was further addressed by a recent cadaver study by Oh et al. The authors found that it was necessary for a rotator cuff tear to include the entire supraspinatus and one-half of the infraspinatus to result in superior and posterior migration of the humeral head. This finding was in agreement with that of most other authors and reemphasizes the necessity of force coupling for the stabilization that allows the shoulder to function. This study was unique in that the superficial shoulder muscles were left intact, and they found that the head was stabilized by activation of the pectoralis major and latissimus dorsi [164, 182, 186–188]. A similar cadaver study by Hansen et al., in which the humeral head was stabilized, demonstrated that increasing force in the remaining cuff muscles and a less significant increase at the deltoid were required to abduct the arm, but that at least until the tear was 7 cm in length, this increased force requirement was well within the physiological range an average person could generate in vivo [71]. Interestingly, this study also showed that massive rotator cuff tears increased the force requirements for the remaining musculature, most notably at the initiation of abduction. For the largest 8 cm tears, the force required was beyond what the deltoid could likely generate in a fatigued state [71].

It is important to note that the aforementioned cadaveric studies are limited by the fact that even when fatigue is factored in, the studies do not take into account the significant pain patients often experience, which may limit muscle activation.

Such pain can cause a reflex inhibition of the cuff musculature that could change shoulder biomechanics. Thus, even small tears can alter shoulder biomechanics in vivo, despite models suggesting that the effect should be minimal. Kelly and colleagues performed a study that compared patients with symptomatic and asymptomatic cuff tears (determined by pain level and range of motion after tear confirmed on MRI) as well as patients with no cuff pathology (determined by MRI). Electromyographical (EMG) analysis of these three patient populations during various functional tests (i.e., internal rotation, lifting weight onto an overhead shelf, etc.) showed statistically significant differences in muscle firing patterns, although sample size was low. The activation of the supraspinatus muscle during all functional tests was greatest in the symptomatic rotator cuff tear patient population and least in the control patient population (no cuff pathology). Asymptomatic patients had an activation level of the supraspinatus muscle that was between that of symptomatic and control patients [190].

Other factors not considered in most biomechanical studies include the fact that chronic tears also develop tendon retraction and fatty infiltration that further decrease the force that a muscle can generate. Those effects may change the pennation angles of individual muscle fibers. These changes can cause further loss of normal shoulder biomechanics [146, 191, 192].

For patients who are poor candidates for rotator cuff repair, physical therapy programs which focus on anterior deltoid strengthening have produced some success in increasing shoulder elev   n and abduction and reducing pain. These   grams focus on the anterior deltoid and the   minor which together may reapproximate for   pling. Furthermore, the anterior portion o   eltoid allows elevation without the shearin   t that activation of the middle portion of th   d may cause [193, 194]. While these studi   est that physical rehabilitation focused on   thening the remaining musculature may al   rly and low demand patient to maintain qu   mal biomechanics, they are likely not a   establish the stabilizing effect of the in   ator cuff, especially in very large rotator c

Summary

The development of rotator cuff pathology is multifactorial in nature; resulting from a combination of intrinsic and extrinsic factors. Age-related degeneration, oxidative stress, vascular changes, and inflammation are all potential contributors to the intrinsic pathology of the rotator cuff. Of the variety of cellular and morphologic changes that are observed in the setting of massive rotator cuff tears, two changes—muscle atrophy and fatty degeneration—are strongly correlated with high repair failure rates and worsening functional outcomes. Yet, the precise molecular basis for these changes is largely unknown.

Massive tears of the rotator cuff prevent the cuff from stabilizing the humeral head on the glenoid to allow other muscles to generate motion across the joint. It is unclear exactly how large a tear must be to cause a loss of the force coupling effect of the rotator cuff and normal shoulder biomechanics. Another major question, still unanswered, is the mechanism behind the evolution of subjective pain in the setting of rotator cuff pathology as many cuff tears are asymptomatic. Investigation and further understanding of these fundamental mechanisms will not only lead to better diagnostic and prognostic capabilities but will also aid in the development of better treatment modalities and adjunctive therapies for massive rotator cuff tears.

References

1. Oh LS, Wolf BR, Hall MP, Levy BA, Marx RG. Indications for rotator cuff repair: a systematic review. Clin Orthop Relat Res. 2007;455:52–63.
2. Bedi A, Dines J, Warren RF, Dines DM. Massive tears of the rotator cuff. J Bone Joint Surg Am. 2010;92:1894–908.
3. Cofield RH, Parvizi J, Hoffmeyer PJ, Lanzer WL, Ilstrup DM, Rowland CM. Surgical repair of chronic rotator cuff tears. A prospective long-term study. J Bone Joint Surg Am. 2001;83-A:71–7.
4. Gerber C, Fuchs B, Hodler J. The results of repair of massive tears of the rotator cuff. J Bone Joint Surg Am. 2000;82:505–15.
5. Burkhart SS. Arthroscopic treatment of massive rotator cuff tears. Clinical results and biomechanical rationale. Clin Orthop Relat Res. 1991;(265):45–56.
6. Harryman 2nd DT, Hettrich CM, Smith KL, Campbell B, Sidles JA, Matsen 3rd FA. A prospective multipractice investigation of patients with full-thickness rotator cuff tears: the importance of comorbidities, practice, and other covariables on self-assessed shoulder function and health status. J Bone Joint Surg Am. 2003;85-A:690–6.
7. Habermeyer P, Krieter C, Tang KL, Lichtenberg S, Magosch P. A new arthroscopic classification of articular-sided supraspinatus footprint lesions: a prospective comparison with Snyder's and Ellman's classification. J Shoulder Elbow Surg. 2008;17:909–13.
8. Ellman H, Kay SP, Wirth M. Arthroscopic treatment of full-thickness rotator cuff tears: 2- to 7-year follow-up study. Arthroscopy. 1993;9:195–200.
9. Ellman H, Hanker G, Bayer M. Repair of the rotator cuff. End-result study of factors influencing reconstruction. J Bone Joint Surg Am. 1986;68:1136–44.
10. Kreuz PC, Remiger A, Erggelet C, Hinterwimmer S, Niemeyer P, Gachter A. Isolated and combined tears of the subscapularis tendon. Am J Sports Med. 2005;33:1831–7.
11. Goutallier D, Postel JM, Gleyze P, Leguilloux P, Van Driessche S. Influence of cuff muscle fatty degeneration on anatomic and functional outcomes after simple suture of full-thickness tears. J Shoulder Elbow Surg. 2003;12:550–4.
12. Smith JG. The classic: pathological appearances of seven cases of injury of the shoulder-joint: with remarks. 1834. Clin Orthop Relat Res. 2010;468:1471–5.
13. Jarjavay JF. Sur la luxation du tendon de la longue portion du muscle biceps humeral; sur la luxation des tendons des muscles peroniers lateraux. Gazette Hebdomadaire de Médecine et de Chir. 1867;21:325.
14. Mclaughlin H, McLaughlin HL, Asherman EG. Lesions of the musculotendinous cuff of the shoulder IV: some observations based upon the results of surgical repair. J Bone Joint Surg. 1951;33:76–86.
15. Armstrong JR. Excision of the acromion in treatment of the supraspinatus syndrome; report of 95 excisions. J Bone Joint Surg Br. 1949;31B:436–42.
16. Watson-Jones R. The classic: "Fractures and Joint Injuries" by Sir Reginald Watson-Jones, taken from "Fractures and Joint Injuries," by R. Watson-Jones, Vol. II, 4th ed., Baltimore, Williams and Wilkins Company, 1955. Clin Orthop Relat Res. 1974;(105):4–10.
17. Mosely H. Shoulder lesions. Edinburgh: F & S Livingstone; 1969.
18. S-P MN. Useful surgical procedures for rheumatoid arthritis involving joints of the upper extremity. Arch Surg. 1943;46:764–70.
19. Codman EA. The shoulder; rupture of the supraspinatus tendon and other lesions in or about the subacromial bursa. Boston: T. Todd company; 1934.
20. Matsen FA. The shoulder. In: Rockwood CAM, Frederick A, editors. Philadelphia: Saunders Elsevier; 2009.
21. Meyer AW. Use destruction in the human body. Cal West Med. 1937;47:375–83.

22. Neer CS. Impingement lesions. Clin Orthop Relat Res. 1983;173:70–7.

23. Neer 2nd CS. Anterior acromioplasty for the chronic impingement syndrome in the shoulder: a preliminary report. J Bone Joint Surg Am. 1972;54:41–50.

24. Bigliani LU, Ticker JB, Flatow EL, Soslowsky LJ, Mow VC. Relationship of acromial architecture and diseases of the rotator cuff. Orthopade. 1991;20: 302–9.

25. Mehta S, Gimbel JA, Soslowsky LJ. Etiologic and pathogenetic factors for rotator cuff tendinopathy. Clin Sports Med. 2003;22:791–812.

26. Uhthoff HK, Hammond DI, Sarkar K, Hooper GJ, Papoff WJ. The role of the coracoacromial ligament in the impingement syndrome. A clinical, radiological and histological study. Int Orthop. 1988;12:97–104.

27. Mayerhoefer ME, Breitenseher MJ, Wurnig C, Roposch A. Shoulder impingement: relationship of clinical symptoms and imaging criteria. Clin J Sport Med. 2009;19:83–9.

28. Ozaki J, Fujimoto S, Nakagawa Y, Masuhara K, Tamai S. Tears of the rotator cuff of the shoulder associated with pathological changes in the acromion. A study in cadavera. J Bone Joint Surg Am. 1988;70:1224–30.

29. Nakajima T, Rokuuma N, Hamada K, Tomatsu T, Fukuda H. Histologic and biomechanical characteristics of the supraspinatus tendon: reference to rotator cuff tearing. J Shoulder Elbow Surg. 1994;3:79–87.

30. Worland RL, Lee D, Orozco CG, SozaRex F, Keenan J. Correlation of age, acromial morphology, and rotator cuff tear pathology diagnosed by ultrasound in asymptomatic patients. J South Orthop Assoc. 2003;12:23–6.

31. Ogata S, Uhthoff HK. Acromial enthesopathy and rotator cuff tear. A radiologic and histologic postmortem investigation of the coracoacromial arch. Clin Orthop Relat Res. 1990;254:39–48.

32. Reilly P, Amis AA, Wallace AL, Emery RJ. Mechanical factors in the initiation and propagation of tears of the rotator cuff. Quantification of strains of the supraspinatus tendon in vitro. J Bone Joint Surg Br. 2003;85:594–9.

33. Edelson G, Teitz C. Internal impingement in the shoulder. J Shoulder Elbow Surg. 2000;9:308–15.

34. Soslowsky LJ, Thomopoulos S, Esmail A, et al. Rotator cuff tendinosis in an animal model: role of extrinsic and overuse factors. Ann Biomed Eng. 2002;30:1057–63.

35. Nho SJ, Yadav H, Shindle MK, Macgillivray JD. Rotator cuff degeneration: etiology and pathogenesis. Am J Sports Med. 2008;36:987–93.

36. Tempelhof S, Rupp S, Seil R. Age-related prevalence of rotator cuff tears in asymptomatic shoulders. J Shoulder Elbow Surg. 1999;8:296–9.

37. Hashimoto T, Nobuhara K, Hamada T. Pathologic evidence of degeneration as a primary cause of rotator cuff tear. Clin Orthop Relat Res. 2003;(415):111–20.

38. Longo UG, Franceschi F, Ruzzini L, et al. Histopathology of the supraspinatus tendon in rotator cuff tears. Am J Sports Med. 2008;36:533–8.

39. Perry SM, McIlhenny SE, Hoffman MC, Soslowsky LJ. Inflammatory and angiogenic mRNA levels are altered in a supraspinatus tendon overuse animal model. J Shoulder Elbow Surg. 2005;14:79S–83.

40. Yuan J, Murrell GA, Trickett A, Wang MX. Involvement of cytochrome c release and caspase-3 activation in the oxidative stress-induced apoptosis in human tendon fibroblasts. Biochim Biophys Acta. 2003;1641:35–41.

41. Wang F, Murrell GA, Wang MX. Oxidative stress-induced c-Jun N-terminal kinase (JNK) activation in tendon cells upregulates MMP1 mRNA and protein expression. J Orthop Res. 2007;25:378–89.

42. Birkedal-Hansen H, Yamada S, Windsor J, et al. Matrix metalloproteinases. Curr Protoc Cell Biol. 2008; Chapter 10: Unit 10.8.

43. Lo IK, Marchuk LL, Hollinshead R, Hart DA, Frank CB. Matrix metalloproteinase and tissue inhibitor of matrix metalloproteinase mRNA levels are specifically altered in torn rotator cuff tendons. Am J Sports Med. 2004;32:1223–9.

44. Magra M, Maffulli N. Matrix metalloproteases: a role in overuse tendinopathies. Br J Sports Med. 2005;39:789–91.

45. Gotoh M, Hamada K, Yamakawa H, Tomonaga A, Inoue A, Fukuda H. Significance of granulation tissue in torn supraspinatus insertions: an immunohistochemical study with antibodies against interleukin-1 beta, cathepsin D, and matrix metalloprotease-1. J Orthop Res. 1997;15:33–9.

46. Rodeo SA, Kawamura S, Kim HJ, Dynybil C, Ying L. Tendon healing in a bone tunnel differs at the tunnel entrance versus the tunnel exit: an effect of graft-tunnel motion? Am J Sports Med. 2006;34: 1790–800.

47. Astrom M, Rausing A. Chronic Achilles tendinopathy. A survey of surgical and histopathologic findings. Clin Orthop Relat Res. 1995;(316):151–64.

48. Maffulli N, Wong J, Almekinders LC. Types and epidemiology of tendinopathy. Clin Sports Med. 2003;22:675–92.

49. Fu SC, Wang W, Pau HM, Wong YP, Chan KM, Rolf CG. Increased expression of transforming growth factor-beta1 in patellar tendinosis. Clin Orthop Relat Res. 2002;(400):174–83.

50. Millar NL, Wei AQ, Molloy TJ, Bonar F, M[...] GA. Cytokines and apoptosis in supraspinatu[...] nopathy. J Bone Joint Surg Br. 2009;91:417[...]

51. Tsuzaki M, Guyton G, Garrett W, et al. I[...] induces COX2, MMP-1, −3 and −13, ADA[...] IL-1 beta and IL-6 in human tendon cells. [...] Res. 2003;21:256–64.

52. Yang G, Im HJ, Wang JH. Repetitive m[...] stretching modulates IL-1beta induced [...] MMP-1 expression, and PGE2 production [...] patellar tendon fibroblasts. Gene. [...] 166–72.

53. Kannus P, Jozsa L. Histopathological cha[...] ceding spontaneous rupture of a tendon. A [...] study of 891 patients. J Bone Joint Surg [...] 73:1507–25.

54. Khan KM, Cook JL, Bonar F, Harcourt P, Astrom M. Histopathology of common tendinopathies. Update and implications for clinical management. Sports Med. 1999;27:393–408.

55. Uhthoff HK, Sano H. Pathology of failure of the rotator cuff tendon. Orthop Clin North Am. 1997;28:31–41.

56. Millar NL, Hueber AJ, Reilly JH, et al. Inflammation is present in early human tendinopathy. Am J Sports Med. 2010;38:2085–91.

57. Lohr JF, Uhthoff HK. The microvascular pattern of the supraspinatus tendon. Clin Orthop Relat Res. 1990;(254):35–8.

58. Miniaci A, Dowdy PA, Willits KR, Vellet AD. Magnetic resonance imaging evaluation of the rotator cuff tendons in the asymptomatic shoulder. Am J Sports Med. 1995;23:142–5.

59. Rudzki JR, Adler RS, Warren RF, et al. Contrast-enhanced ultrasound characterization of the vascularity of the rotator cuff tendon: age- and activity-related changes in the intact asymptomatic rotator cuff. J Shoulder Elbow Surg. 2008;17:96S–100.

60. Rathbun JB, Macnab I. The microvascular pattern of the rotator cuff. J Bone Joint Surg Br. 1970;52:540–53.

61. Brooks CH, Revell WJ, Heatley FW. A quantitative histological study of the vascularity of the rotator cuff tendon. J Bone Joint Surg Br. 1992;74:151–3.

62. Benson RT, McDonnell SM, Knowles HJ, Rees JL, Carr AJ, Hulley PA. Tendinopathy and tears of the rotator cuff are associated with hypoxia and apoptosis. J Bone Joint Surg Br. 2010;92:448–53.

63. Baumgarten KM, Gerlach D, Galatz LM, et al. Cigarette smoking increases the risk for rotator cuff tears. Clin Orthop Relat Res. 2010;468:1534–41.

64. Abboud JA, Kim JS. The effect of hypercholesterolemia on rotator cuff disease. Clin Orthop Relat Res. 2010;468:1493–7.

65. Chaudhury S, Carr AJ. Lessons we can learn from gene expression patterns in rotator cuff tears and tendinopathies. J Shoulder Elbow Surg. 2012;21:191–9.

66. Lippi G, Longo UG, Maffulli N. Genetics and sports. Br Med Bull. 2010;93:27–47.

67. Longo UG, Lamberti A, Maffulli N, Denaro V. Tendon augmentation grafts: a systematic review. Br Med Bull. 2010;94:165–88.

68. Longo UG, Lamberti A, Maffulli N, Denaro V. Tissue engineered biological augmentation for tendon healing: a systematic review. Br Med Bull. 2011;98:31–59.

69. Harvie P, Ostlere SJ, Teh J, et al. Genetic influences in the aetiology of tears of the rotator cuff. Sibling risk of a full-thickness tear. J Bone Joint Surg Br. 2004;86:696–700.

70. Molloy TJ, Kemp MW, Wang Y, Murrell GA. Microarray analysis of the tendinopathic rat supraspinatus tendon: glutamate signaling and its potential role in tendon degeneration. J Appl Physiol. 2006;101:1702–9.

71. Rees JD, Wilson AM, Wolman RL. Current concepts in the management of tendon disorders. Rheumatology (Oxford). 2006;45:508–21.

72. Hart DA Frank CB, Bray RC. Inflammatory processes in repetitive motion and overuse syndromes: potential role of neurogenic mechanisms in tendons and ligaments. In: Gordon SL, Blair SJ, Fine LJ, National Institute of Arthritis and Musculoskeletal and Skin Diseases (U.S.), editors. Repetitive motion disorders of the upper extremity. 1st ed. Rosemont: American Academy of Orthopaedic Surgeons; 1995, xxii, 565 p.

73. Gotoh M, Hamada K, Yamakawa H, Inoue A, Fukuda H. Increased substance P in subacromial bursa and shoulder pain in rotator cuff diseases. J Orthop Res. 1998;16:618–21.

74. Yamaguchi K, Tetro AM, Blam O, Evanoff BA, Teefey SA, Middleton WD. Natural history of asymptomatic rotator cuff tears: a longitudinal analysis of asymptomatic tears detected sonographically. J Shoulder Elbow Surg. 2001;10:199–203.

75. Yamaguchi K, Ditsios K, Middleton WD, Hildebolt CF, Galatz LM, Teefey SA. The demographic and morphological features of rotator cuff disease. A comparison of asymptomatic and symptomatic shoulders. J Bone Joint Surg Am. 2006;88:1699–704.

76. Gotoh M, Hamada K, Yamakawa H, et al. Interleukin-1-induced glenohumeral synovitis and shoulder pain in rotator cuff diseases. J Orthop Res. 2002;20:1365–71.

77. Meyer DC, Hoppeler H, von Rechenberg B, Gerber C. A pathomechanical concept explains muscle loss and fatty muscular changes following surgical tendon release. J Orthop Res. 2004;22:1004–7.

78. Itoigawa Y, Kishimoto KN, Sano H, Kaneko K, Itoi E. Molecular mechanism of fatty degeneration in rotator cuff muscle with tendon rupture. J Orthop Res. 2011;29:861–6.

79. Chaudhury S, Dines JS, Delos D, Warren RF, Voigt C, Rodeo SA. Role of fatty infiltration in the pathophysiology and outcomes of rotator cuff tears. Arthritis Care Res (Hoboken). 2012;64:76–82.

80. Steinbacher P, Tauber M, Kogler S, Stoiber W, Resch H, Sanger AM. Effects of rotator cuff ruptures on the cellular and intracellular composition of the human supraspinatus muscle. Tissue Cell. 2010;42:37–41.

81. Melis B, DeFranco MJ, Chuinard C, Walch G. Natural history of fatty infiltration and atrophy of the supraspinatus muscle in rotator cuff tears. Clin Orthop Relat Res. 2010;468:1498–505.

82. Nakagaki K, Ozaki J, Tomita Y, Tamai S. Fatty degeneration in the supraspinatus muscle after rotator cuff tear. J Shoulder Elbow Surg. 1996;5:194–200.

83. Kim HM, Dahiya N, Teefey SA, Keener JD, Galatz LM, Yamaguchi K. Relationship of tear size and location to fatty degeneration of the rotator cuff. J Bone Joint Surg Am. 2010;92:829–39.

84. Kim HM, Galatz LM, Lim C, Havlioglu N, Thomopoulos S. The effect of tear size and nerve

injury on rotator cuff muscle fatty degeneration in a rodent animal model. J Shoulder Elbow Surg. 2012;21:847–58.

85. Liu X, Laron D, Natsuhara K, Manzano G, Kim HT, Feeley BT. A mouse model of massive rotator cuff tears. J Bone Joint Surg Am. 2012;94:e41.

86. Liu X, Manzano G, Kim HT, Feeley BT. A rat model of massive rotator cuff tears. J Orthop Res. 2011;29:588–95.

87. Mallon WJ, Wilson RJ, Basamania CJ. The association of suprascapular neuropathy with massive rotator cuff tears: a preliminary report. J Shoulder Elbow Surg. 2006;15:395–8.

88. Rowshan K, Hadley S, Pham K, Caiozzo V, Lee TQ, Gupta R. Development of fatty atrophy after neurologic and rotator cuff injuries in an animal model of rotator cuff pathology. J Bone Joint Surg Am. 2010;92:2270–8.

89. Shah AA, Butler RB, Sung SY, Wells JH, Higgins LD, Warner JJ. Clinical outcomes of suprascapular nerve decompression. J Shoulder Elbow Surg. 2011;20:975–82.

90. Gladstone JN, Bishop JY, Lo IK, Flatow EL. Fatty infiltration and atrophy of the rotator cuff do not improve after rotator cuff repair and correlate with poor functional outcome. Am J Sports Med. 2007;35:719–28.

91. Rubino LJ, Sprott DC, Stills Jr HF, Crosby LA. Fatty infiltration does not progress after rotator cuff repair in a rabbit model. Arthroscopy. 2008;24:936–40.

92. Yamaguchi H, Suenaga N, Oizumi N, Hosokawa Y, Kanaya F. Will preoperative atrophy and Fatty degeneration of the shoulder muscles improve after rotator cuff repair in patients with massive rotator cuff tears? Adv Orthop. 2012;2012:195876.

93. Goutallier D, Postel JM, Bernageau J, Lavau L, Voisin MC. Fatty muscle degeneration in cuff ruptures. Pre- and postoperative evaluation by CT scan. Clin Orthop Relat Res. 1994;(304):78–83.

94. Mellado JM, Calmet J, Olona M, et al. Surgically repaired massive rotator cuff tears: MRI of tendon integrity, muscle fatty degeneration, and muscle atrophy correlated with intraoperative and clinical findings. AJR Am J Roentgenol. 2005;184: 1456–63.

95. Laron D, Samagh SP, Liu X, Kim HT, Feeley BT. Muscle degeneration in rotator cuff tears. J Shoulder Elbow Surg. 2012;21:164–74.

96. Senf SM, Dodd SL, Judge AR. FOXO signaling is required for disuse muscle atrophy and is directly regulated by Hsp70. Am J Physiol Cell Physiol. 2010;298:C38–45.

97. Senf SM, Dodd SL, McClung JM, Judge AR. Hsp70 overexpression inhibits NF-kappaB and Foxo3a transcriptional activities and prevents skeletal muscle atrophy. FASEB J. 2008;22:3836–45.

98. Schmutz S, Fuchs T, Regenfelder F, Steinmann P, Zumstein M, Fuchs B. Expression of atrophy mRNA relates to tendon tear size in supraspinatus muscle. Clin Orthop Relat Res. 2009;467:457–64.

99. Liu X, et al. Evaluation of Akt/mTOR activity in muscle atrophy after rotator cuff tears in a rat model. J Orthop Res. 2012;30:1440–6.

100. Perry RL, Rudnick MA. Molecular mechanisms regulating myogenic determination and differentiation. Front Biosci. 2000;5:D750–67.

101. Sabourin LA, Rudnicki MA. The molecular regulation of myogenesis. Clin Genet. 2000;57:16–25.

102. Otto TC, Lane MD. Adipose development: from stem cell to adipocyte. Crit Rev Biochem Mol Biol. 2005;40:229–42.

103. Rosen ED, Walkey CJ, Puigserver P, Spiegelman BM. Transcriptional regulation of adipogenesis. Genes Dev. 2000;14:1293–307.

104. Frey E, Regenfelder F, Sussmann P, et al. Adipogenic and myogenic gene expression in rotator cuff muscle of the sheep after tendon tear. J Orthop Res. 2009;27:504–9.

105. Bennett CN, Hodge CL, MacDougald OA, Schwartz J. Role of Wnt10b and C/EBPalpha in spontaneous adipogenesis of 243 cells. Biochem Biophys Res Commun. 2003;302:12–6.

106. Itoigawa Y, Kishimoto KN, Okuno H, Sano H, Kaneko K, Itoi E. Hypoxia induces adipogenic differentiation of myoblastic cell lines. Biochem Biophys Res Commun. 2010;399:721–6.

107. Park JR, Jung JW, Lee YS, Kang KS. The roles of Wnt antagonists Dkk1 and sFRP4 during adipogenesis of human adipose tissue-derived mesenchymal stem cells. Cell Prolif. 2008;41:859–74.

108. Safran O, Derwin KA, Powell K, Iannotti JP. Changes in rotator cuff muscle volume, fat content, and passive mechanics after chronic detachment in a canine model. J Bone Joint Surg Am. 2005;87: 2662–70.

109. Akimoto T, Ushida T, Miyaki S, et al. Mechanical stretch inhibits myoblast-to-adipocyte differentiation through Wnt signaling. Biochem Biophys Res Commun. 2005;329:381–5.

110. Lakemeier S, Reichelt JJ, Patzer T, Fuchs-Winkelmann S, Paletta JR, Schofer MD. The association between retraction of the torn rotator cuff and increasing expression of hypoxia inducible factor 1alpha and vascular endothelial growth factor expression: an immunohistological study. BMC Musculoskelet Disord. 2010;11:230.

111. Woo SL, An K-N, Arnoczky SP, et al. Anatomy, biology, and biomechanics of tendon, ligament, and meniscus. In: Simon SR, American Academy of Orthopaedic Surgeons, editors. Orthopaedic basic science. Rosemont: American Academy of Orthopaedic Surgeons; 1994, xvi, 704 p.

112. Bedi A, Maak T, Walsh C, et al. Cytokines in rotator cuff degeneration and repair. J Shoulder Elbow Surg. 2012;21:218–27.

113. Gulotta LV, Rodeo SA. Growth factors for rotator cuff repair. Clin Sports Med. 2009;28:13–23.

114. Montgomery SR, Petrigliano FA, Gamradt SC. Failed rotator cuff surgery, evaluation and decision making. Clin Sports Med. 2012;31:693–712.

115. Gamradt SC, Gallo RA, Adler RS, et al. Vascularity of the supraspinatus tendon three months after repair: characterization using contrast-enhanced ultrasound. J Shoulder Elbow Surg. 2010;19:73–80.

116. Gerber C, Schneeberger AG, Perren SM, Nyffeler RW. Experimental rotator cuff repair. A preliminary study. J Bone Joint Surg Am. 1999;81:1281–90.

117. Carpenter JE, Thomopoulos S, Flanagan CL, DeBano CM, Soslowsky LJ. Rotator cuff defect healing: a biomechanical and histologic analysis in an animal model. J Shoulder Elbow Surg. 1998; 7:599–605.

118. Hays PL, Kawamura S, Deng XH, et al. The role of macrophages in early healing of a tendon graft in a bone tunnel. J Bone Joint Surg Am. 2008;90: 565–79.

119. Harwood FL, Goomer RS, Gelberman RH, Silva MJ, Amiel D. Regulation of alpha(v)beta3 and alpha5beta1 integrin receptors by basic fibroblast growth factor and platelet-derived growth factor-BB in intrasynovial flexor tendon cells. Wound Repair Regen. 1999;7:381–8.

120. Nakamura N, Shino K, Natsuume T, et al. Early biological effect of in vivo gene transfer of platelet-derived growth factor (PDGF)-B into healing patellar ligament. Gene Ther. 1998;5:1165–70.

121. Nakamura N, Timmermann SA, Hart DA, et al. A comparison of in vivo gene delivery methods for antisense therapy in ligament healing. Gene Ther. 1998;5:1455–61.

122. Yoshikawa Y, Abrahamsson SO. Dose-related cellular effects of platelet-derived growth factor-BB differ in various types of rabbit tendons in vitro. Acta Orthop Scand. 2001;72:287–92.

123. Hee CK, Dines JS, Dines DM, et al. Augmentation of a rotator cuff suture repair using rhPDGF-BB and a type I bovine collagen matrix in an ovine model. Am J Sports Med. 2011;39:1630–9.

124. Campbell BH, Agarwal C, Wang JH. TGF-beta1, TGF-beta3, and PGE(2) regulate contraction of human patellar tendon fibroblasts. Biomech Model Mechanobiol. 2004;2:239–45.

125. Klein MB, Yalamanchi N, Pham H, Longaker MT, Chang J. Flexor tendon healing in vitro: effects of TGF-beta on tendon cell collagen production. J Hand Surg Am. 2002;27:615–20.

126. Kovacevic D, Fox AJ, Bedi A, et al. Calcium-phosphate matrix with or without TGF-beta3 improves tendon-bone healing after rotator cuff repair. Am J Sports Med. 2011;39:811–9.

127. Wolfman NM, Hattersley G, Cox K, et al. Ectopic induction of tendon and ligament in rats by growth and differentiation factors 5, 6, and 7, members of the TGF-beta gene family. J Clin Invest. 1997; 100:321–30.

128. Abrahamsson SO, Lundborg G, Lohmander LS. Recombinant human insulin-like growth factor-I stimulates in vitro matrix synthesis and cell proliferation in rabbit flexor tendon. J Orthop Res. 1991;9:495–502.

129. Dahlgren LA, van der Meulen MC, Bertram JE, Starrak GS, Nixon AJ. Insulin-like growth factor-I improves cellular and molecular aspects of healing in a collagenase-induced model of flexor tendinitis. J Orthop Res. 2002;20:910–9.

130. Kurtz CA, Loebig TG, Anderson DD, DeMeo PJ, Campbell PG. Insulin-like growth factor I accelerates functional recovery from Achilles tendon injury in a rat model. Am J Sports Med. 1999;27:363–9.

131. Canalis E, Centrella M, McCarthy T. Effects of basic fibroblast growth factor on bone formation in vitro. J Clin Invest. 1988;81:1572–7.

132. Gospodarowicz D, Neufeld G, Schweigerer L. Molecular and biological characterization of fibroblast growth factor, an angiogenic factor which also controls the proliferation and differentiation of mesoderm and neuroectoderm derived cells. Cell Differ. 1986;19:1–17.

133. Ide J, Kikukawa K, Hirose J, et al. The effect of a local application of fibroblast growth factor-2 on tendon-to-bone remodeling in rats with acute injury and repair of the supraspinatus tendon. J Shoulder Elbow Surg. 2009;18:391–8.

134. Chan BP, Chan KM, Maffulli N, Webb S, Lee KK. Effect of basic fibroblast growth factor. An in vitro study of tendon healing. Clin Orthop Relat Res. 1997;(342):239–47.

135. Chan BP, Fu S, Qin L, Lee K, Rolf CG, Chan K. Effects of basic fibroblast growth factor (bFGF) on early stages of tendon healing: a rat patellar tendon model. Acta Orthop Scand. 2000;71:513–8.

136. Takahasih S, Nakajima M, Kobayashi M, et al. Effect of recombinant basic fibroblast growth factor (bFGF) on fibroblast-like cells from human rotator cuff tendon. Tohoku J Exp Med. 2002; 198:207–14.

137. Tang JB, Cao Y, Zhu B, Xin KQ, Wang XT, Liu PY. Adeno-associated virus-2-mediated bFGF gene transfer to digital flexor tendons significantly increases healing strength: an in vivo study. J Bone Joint Surg Am. 2008;90:1078–89.

138. Chang J, Most D, Thunder R, Mehrara B, Longaker MT, Lineaweaver WC. Molecular studies in flexor tendon wound healing: the role of basic fibroblast growth factor gene expression. J Hand Surg Am. 1998;23:1052–8.

139. Khan U, Occleston NL, Khaw PT, McGrouther DA. Differences in proliferative rate and collagen lattice contraction between endotenon and synovial fibroblasts. J Hand Surg Am. 1998;23:266–73.

140. Thomopoulos S, Harwood FL, Silva MJ, Amiel D, Gelberman RH. Effect of several growth factors on canine flexor tendon fibroblast proliferation and collagen synthesis in vitro. J Hand Surg Am. 2005; 30:441–7.

141. Tsuzaki M, Brigman BE, Yamamoto J, et al. Insulin-like growth factor-I is expressed by avian flexor tendon cells. J Orthop Res. 2000;18:546–56.

142. Bidder M, Towler DA, Gelberman RH, Boyer MI. Expression of mRNA for vascular endothelial

growth factor at the repair site of healing canine flexor tendon. J Orthop Res. 2000;18:247–52.

143. Boyer MI, Watson JT, Lou J, Manske PR, Gelberman RH, Cai SR. Quantitative variation in vascular endothelial growth factor mRNA expression during early flexor tendon healing: an investigation in a canine model. J Orthop Res. 2001;19:869–72.

144. Petersen W, Pufe T, Unterhauser F, Zantop T, Mentlein R, Weiler A. The splice variants 120 and 164 of the angiogenic peptide vascular endothelial cell growth factor (VEGF) are expressed during Achilles tendon healing. Arch Orthop Trauma Surg. 2003;123:475–80.

145. Petersen W, Unterhauser F, Pufe T, Zantop T, Sudkamp NP, Weiler A. The angiogenic peptide vascular endothelial growth factor (VEGF) is expressed during the remodeling of free tendon grafts in sheep. Arch Orthop Trauma Surg. 2003;123:168–74.

146. Hersche O, Gerber C. Passive tension in the supraspinatus musculotendinous unit after long-standing rupture of its tendon: a preliminary report. J Shoulder Elbow Surg. 1998;7:393–6.

147. Gerber C, Schneeberger AG, Hoppeler H, Meyer DC. Correlation of atrophy and fatty infiltration on strength and integrity of rotator cuff repairs: a study in thirteen patients. J Shoulder Elbow Surg. 2007;16:691–6.

148. Liem D, Lichtenberg S, Magosch P, Habermeyer P. Magnetic resonance imaging of arthroscopic supraspinatus tendon repair. J Bone Joint Surg Am. 2007;89:1770–6.

149. Coleman SH, Fealy S, Ehteshami JR, et al. Chronic rotator cuff injury and repair model in sheep. J Bone Joint Surg Am. 2003;85-A:2391–402.

150. Bassett RW, Cofield RH. Acute tears of the rotator cuff. The timing of surgical repair. Clin Orthop Relat Res. 1983;(175):18–24.

151. Boileau P, Brassart N, Watkinson DJ, Carles M, Hatzidakis AM, Krishnan SG. Arthroscopic repair of full-thickness tears of the supraspinatus: does the tendon really heal? J Bone Joint Surg Am. 2005;87:1229–40.

152. Cole BJ, McCarty 3rd LP, Kang RW, Alford W, Lewis PB, Hayden JK. Arthroscopic rotator cuff repair: prospective functional outcome and repair integrity at minimum 2-year follow-up. J Shoulder Elbow Surg. 2007;16:579–85.

153. DeFranco MJ, Bershadsky B, Ciccone J, Yum JK, Iannotti JP. Functional outcome of arthroscopic rotator cuff repairs: a correlation of anatomic and clinical results. J Shoulder Elbow Surg. 2007;16:759–65.

154. Gazielly DF, Gleyze P, Montagnon C. Functional and anatomical results after rotator cuff repair. Clin Orthop Relat Res. 1994;(304):43–53.

155. Harryman 2nd DT, Mack LA, Wang KY, Jackins SE, Richardson ML, Matsen 3rd FA. Repairs of the rotator cuff. Correlation of functional results with integrity of the cuff. J Bone Joint Surg Am. 1991;73:982–9.

156. Keener JD, Wei AS, Kim HM, et al. Revision arthroscopic rotator cuff repair: repair integrity and clinical outcome. J Bone Joint Surg Am. 2010;92:590–8.

157. Nho SJ, Brown BS, Lyman S, Adler RS, Altchek DW, MacGillivray JD. Prospective analysis of arthroscopic rotator cuff repair: prognostic factors affecting clinical and ultrasound outcome. J Shoulder Elbow Surg. 2009;18:13–20.

158. Cohen DB, Kawamura S, Ehteshami JR, Rodeo SA. Indomethacin and celecoxib impair rotator cuff tendon-to-bone healing. Am J Sports Med. 2006;34:362–9.

159. An KN, Chao EY. Kinematic analysis of human movement. Ann Biomed Eng. 1984;12:585–97.

160. Hansen ML, Otis JC, Johnson JS, Cordasco FA, Craig EV, Warren RF. Biomechanics of massive rotator cuff tears: implications for treatment. J Bone Joint Surg Am. 2008;90:316–25.

161. Itoi E. Biomechanics of the shoulder. In: Rockwood C, Matsen F, editors. The shoulder. Philadelphia: Saunders Elsevier; 2009.

162. Bechtol CO. Biomechanics of the shoulder. Clin Orthop Relat Res. 1980:37–41.

163. Markhede G, Monastyrski J, Stener B. Shoulder function after deltoid muscle removal. Acta Orthop Scand. 1985;56:242–4.

164. Thompson WO, Debski RE, Boardman 3rd ND, et al. A biomechanical analysis of rotator cuff deficiency in a cadaveric model. Am J Sports Med. 1996;24:286–92.

165. Itoi E, Minagawa H, Sato T, Sato K, Tabata S. Isokinetic strength after tears of the supraspinatus tendon. J Bone Joint Surg Br. 1997;79:77–82.

166. Kuechle DK, Newman SR, Itoi E, Niebur GL, Morrey BF, An KN. The relevance of the moment arm of shoulder muscles with respect to axial rotation of the glenohumeral joint in four positions. Clin Biomech (Bristol, Avon). 2000;15:322–9.

167. Howell SM, Imobersteg AM, Seger DH, Marone PJ. Clarification of the role of the supraspinatus muscle in shoulder function. J Bone Joint Surg Am. 1986;68:398–404.

168. Sharkey NA, Marder RA, Hanson PB. The entire rotator cuff contributes to elevation of the arm. J Orthop Res. 1994;12:699–708.

169. O'Brien SJ, Schwartz RS, Warren RF, Torzilli PA. Capsular restraints to anterior-posterior motion of the abducted shoulder: a biomechanical study. J Shoulder Elbow Surg. 1995;4:298–308.

170. Kumar VP, Balasubramaniam P. The role of atmospheric pressure in stabilising the shoulder. An experimental study. J Bone Joint Surg Br. 1985;67:719–21.

171. Gibb TD, Sidles JA, Harryman 2nd DT, McQuade KJ, Matsen 3rd FA. The effect of capsular venting on glenohumeral laxity. Clin Orthop Relat Res. 1991;(268):120–7.

172. Howell SM, Kraft TA. The role of the supraspinatus and infraspinatus muscles in glenohumeral kinematics of anterior should instability. Clin Orthop Relat Res. 1991;(263):128–34.

173. Turkel SJ, Panio MW, Marshall JL, Girgis FG. Stabilizing mechanisms preventing anterior dislocation of the glenohumeral joint. J Bone Joint Surg Am. 1981;63:1208–17.

174. Longo UG, Berton A, Papapietro N, Maffulli N, Denaro V. Biomechanics of the rotator cuff: European perspective. Med Sport Sci. 2012;57:10–7.

175. Inman VT, Saunders JB, Abbott LC. Observations of the function of the shoulder joint. Clin Orthop Relat Res. 1944;1996:3–12.

176. Saha AK. Dynamic stability of the glenohumeral joint. Acta Orthop Scand. 1971;42:491–505.

177. Kido T, Itoi E, Konno N, Sano A, Urayama M, Sato K. The depressor function of biceps on the head of the humerus in shoulders with tears of the rotator cuff. J Bone Joint Surg Br. 2000;82:416–9.

178. Parsons IM, Apreleva M, Fu FH, Woo SL. The effect of rotator cuff tears on reaction forces at the glenohumeral joint. J Orthop Res. 2002;20:439–46.

179. Poppen NK, Walker PS. Forces at the glenohumeral joint in abduction. Clin Orthop Relat Res. 1978;(135):165–70.

180. Yanagawa T, Goodwin CJ, Shelburne KB, Giphart JE, Torry MR, Pandy MG. Contributions of the individual muscles of the shoulder to glenohumeral joint stability during abduction. J Biomech Eng. 2008;130:021024.

181. David G, Magarey ME, Jones MA, Dvir Z, Turker KS, Sharpe M. EMG and strength correlates of selected shoulder muscles during rotations of the glenohumeral joint. Clin Biomech (Bristol, Avon). 2000;15:95–102.

182. Oh JH, Jun BJ, McGarry MH, Lee TQ. Does a critical rotator cuff tear stage exist?: a biomechanical study of rotator cuff tear progression in human cadaver shoulders. J Bone Joint Surg Am. 2011;93:2100–9.

183. Mall NA, Kim HM, Keener JD, et al. Symptomatic progression of asymptomatic rotator cuff tears: a prospective study of clinical and sonographic variables. J Bone Joint Surg Am. 2010;92:2623–33.

184. McMahon PJ, Debski RE, Thompson WO, Warner JJ, Fu FH, Woo SL. Shoulder muscle forces and tendon excursions during glenohumeral abduction in the scapular plane. J Shoulder Elbow Surg. 1995;4:199–208.

185. Graichen H, Stammberger T, Bonel H, Karl-Hans E, Reiser M, Eckstein F. Glenohumeral translation during active and passive elevation of the shoulder – a 3D open-MRI study. J Biomech. 2000;33:609–13.

186. Burkhart SS, Nottage WM, Ogilvie-Harris DJ, Kohn HS, Pachelli A. Partial repair of irreparable rotator cuff tears. Arthroscopy. 1994;10:363–70.

187. Gartsman GM. Massive, irreparable tears of the rotator cuff. Results of operative debridement and subacromial decompression. J Bone Joint Surg Am. 1997;79:715–21.

188. Su WR, Budoff JE, Luo ZP. The effect of anterosuperior rotator cuff tears on glenohumeral translation. Arthroscopy. 2009;25:282–9.

189. Burkhart SS. Fluoroscopic comparison of kinematic patterns in massive rotator cuff tears. A suspension bridge model. Clin Orthop Relat Res. 1992;(284):144–52.

190. Kelly BT, Williams RJ, Cordasco FA, et al. Differential patterns of muscle activation in patients with symptomatic and asymptomatic rotator cuff tears. J Shoulder Elbow Surg. 2005;14:165–71.

191. Warner JJ. Management of massive irreparable rotator cuff tears: the role of tendon transfer. Instr Course Lect. 2001;50:63–71.

192. Burkhart SS, Barth JR, Richards DP, Zlatkin MB, Larsen M. Arthroscopic repair of massive rotator cuff tears with stage 3 and 4 fatty degeneration. Arthroscopy. 2007;23:347–54.

193. Ainsworth R. Physiotherapy rehabilitation in patients with massive, irreparable rotator cuff tears. Musculoskeletal Care. 2006;4:140–51.

194. Levy O, Mullett H, Roberts S, Copeland S. The role of anterior deltoid reeducation in patients with massive irreparable degenerative rotator cuff tears. J Shoulder Elbow Surg. 2008;17:863–70.

History and Physical Exam

2

Lawrence V. Gulotta

Pearls and Pitfalls

Pearls

- It is important to determine if the patient's primary complaint is pain or weakness since treatments may differ.
- Patients may have significant atrophy in the infraspinatus fossa.
- If a patient is unable to actively elevate, an injection of local anesthetic with reexamination can be useful to determine if their weakness is due to pain or a biomechanical imbalance.
- Patients with an external rotation lag with elevation often have difficulty positioning their hands in space in order to perform activities of daily living, such as hair care.

Pittfalls

- Patients with Parsonage-Turner Syndrome, or brachial neuritis, may present similar to a patient with a massive rotator cuff tear and should be considered in the diagnosis.
- Patients with pseudoparalysis due to pain inhibition should make drastic improvements with cortisone and physical therapy, and therefore quick decisions to proceed with surgery should be avoided.
- It is important to examine and document the function of the axillary nerve and the integrity of the deltoid since most treatments will depend on their function in the absence of a functional rotator cuff.

Introduction

The history and physical examination of a patient who presents with a massive rotator cuff tear is arguably the most critical aspect of their evaluation. Most patients can be diagnosed with a large rotator cuff tear based on their history and physical examination alone. As with any subjective data accumulation, the information gleaned from this portion of the evaluation is user dependent. However, accuracy improves with experience. Comfort with the techniques outlined in this chapter is important to be able to accurately diagnose massive rotator cuff tears and develop treatment plans that can most adequately address the patient's concerns.

L.V. Gulotta, MD (✉)
Sports Medicine and Shoulder Service,
Hospital for Special Surgery, 535 E 70th Street,
New York, NY 10021, USA

Department of Orthopedic Surgery,
Weill Cornell Medical School, New York, NY, USA
e-mail: GulottaL@hss.edu

L.V. Gulotta and E.V. Craig (eds.), *Massive Rotator Cuff Tears: Diagnosis and Management*,
DOI 10.1007/978-1-4899-7494-5_2, © Springer Science+Business Media New York 2015

History

The most important information that is gathered from the initial visit is the patient's chief complaint. Patients may complain of pain, weakness, or a combination of both. It is important to delineate which one is the most important to them. This will set forth a treatment algorithm based on why the patient is seeking medical intervention. A patient without any pain who presents solely with weakness should be offered different treatment options than a patient who presents with only pain and no complaints of weakness. Both scenarios are possible, even in patients with massive rotator cuff tears. Patients will often state that both are equally important. In those scenarios, an attempt should be made to have the patient try to choose one or the other. This can be helpful in determining the reason for why the patient is seeking medical care and will help set expectations moving forward.

Once a chief complaint is established, a history of present illness should follow. During this portion of the history, all pertinent information such as duration of symptoms, location and quality of pain, any antecedent trauma, pain at night, and whether radicular symptoms are present can be important in localizing the pathology. Patients may or may not report an antecedent trauma prior to their symptoms. When pressed, patients may state that they did have trauma several years back or initially had pain but then improved. Most patients with massive tears do report a long-standing history of shoulder complaints prior to presentation. The exact location of the pain can be very helpful in determining the pathology present. It is often useful to ask the patient to point with one finger to where the pain is most severe. On occasion, patients will point directly over their acromioclavicular (AC) joint or over their long head of the biceps tendon. This can alert the examiner to pathology at those two structures. While patients may have a massive rotator cuff tear, their symptoms may adequately be treated by recognizing and addressing pathology at the long head of the biceps tendon and the AC joint [1]. Patients may also report that the pain is mostly in the back of their shoulder or into their neck. This should direct the examiner to scapulothoracic or cervical spine issues. This would be particularly true if the patient also complains of radicular symptoms that traverse down the arm.

A very useful question that should be asked of all patients is what they would like to do but cannot do, because of pain and dysfunction of their shoulder. This simple question gets to the heart of why the patient is seeking treatment and what components of their shoulder dysfunction they would like to improve. It also helps set expectations in terms of whether or not these things can reasonably be attained.

A thorough history of any previous treatment on the involved shoulder should be obtained. If the patient has had previous surgeries, operative notes can be helpful to determine exactly what was done. Often, there are discrepancies between the patient and the surgeon's descriptions of what was found and accomplished at the time of surgery. Any history of infection should also be determined. Pertinent issues in the patient's medical history are also important since they may affect rotator cuff healing. In particular, comorbidities such as diabetes, smoking, and autoimmune disease are a poor prognostic indicator of achieving healing following any rotator cuff repair [2–5]. This should be determined in the initial consultation. Also, a history of frequent falls may warn against surgical intervention.

Physical Examination

In order to perform a thorough physical examination, the patient needs to be dressed appropriately. Men are asked to take off their shirts in order to facilitate visual inspection of the shoulder girdle. Women are asked to either wear a tank top or a gown that is placed under both arms, but over the breasts, such that both shoulders can be evaluated.

The physical examination of the shoulder begins by evaluating the patient's cervical spine. The patient is asked to move their head up, and down, and to each side. A Spurling's test is then performed by extending the patient's neck and then moving it from side to side. This maneuver can impinge the nerves in the foramen and recreate radicular pain. Many patients will have pain with neck maneuvers, and it is important to determine if the pain they experience with the examination is the same pain for which they are seeking treatment, or if this is a different pain.

Inspection of the shoulder girdle can yield valuable information. Previous incisions should be inspected for any signs of infection such as erythema, warmth, or swelling. Tone of the deltoid can also be ascertained. This is particularly important if the patient had previous open rotator cuff repairs, as deltoid dehiscence can occur and complicate future treatments. Atrophy of the infraspinatus fossa is a common finding in patients with massive rotator cuff tears and can be easily identified in most patients.

Palpation then follows in a purposeful manner. In particular, it is useful to palpate directly over the AC joint and the long head of the biceps tendon. Throughout the palpation, it is important to compare the contralateral side since deep palpation of any shoulder may cause pain that is not necessarily pathologic. It is also important to determine whether or not the pain the patient experiences during the physical examination is the pain they most commonly experience or if a new pain is being created in response to the examination itself. Tenderness to palpation directly over the AC joint or the long head of the biceps tendon may serve as a guide to direct future treatment options [1]. In patients who were previously in an accident or have ongoing legal disputes present, it can be useful to palpate nonanatomic locations around the shoulder. Exquisite pain to palpation throughout the entire shoulder girdle over nonspecific anatomic areas may indicate either malingering, or a myofascial injury, that may not be amenable to surgical intervention.

Active and passive motion should be evaluated. Active motion is evaluated with the patient being asked to elevate the arms in the scapular plane. Patients are next asked to externally rotate the arms with the elbows at the side and then internally rotate by placing the hand behind the back as far up as they are able to achieve. If a patient has full active range of motion, then there

is no need to test passive range of motion. However, if there is a discrepancy or lack of active range of motion, then passive range of motion should be determined. If the active and passive range of motion are limited and equivalent, then concern should be raised for either arthritis or a frozen shoulder. However, if there is a lag between active and passive range of motion, this can be indicative of a rotator cuff tear. When patients are performing active range of motion, it is important to evaluate the scapula for scapular rhythm. It is also important to identify other compensatory mechanisms such as a shrug or if there is anterosuperior escape present.

Most compensatory mechanisms such as a shrug and scapular dyskinesia can typically be corrected with a targeted physical therapy regimen. However, if frank anterosuperior escape is present, then this is a poor prognostic indicator for eventual arm elevation even with adequate physical therapy [6]. Anterosuperior escape is identified on physical examination by seeing the humeral head becoming more prominent in the anterior deltoid. It becomes quite evident especially in smaller patients that the humeral head is not being contained under the coracoacromial arch. This is typically seen in patients that have involvement of the subscapularis in addition to superior and possibly posterior rotator cuff tears.

The most important thing to determine when performing the physical examination of the patient is whether or not they are able to elevate their arm above horizontal. Patients who are unable to elevate their arm above horizontal in the absence of a nerve injury are considered to have pseudoparalysis [7]. Patients who are able to adequately elevate their arm above their head can typically have enough strength to perform most activities of daily living; however, they usually state that pain is their primary complaint. In patients with pseudoparalysis, it is important to understand whether the inability to elevate is coming from a true biomechanical insufficiency or if it is the result of pain inhibition. In these circumstances, an injection of local anesthetic can be very useful. Typically, this is also combined with cortisone to potentially give the patient some lasting relief as well. After the patient

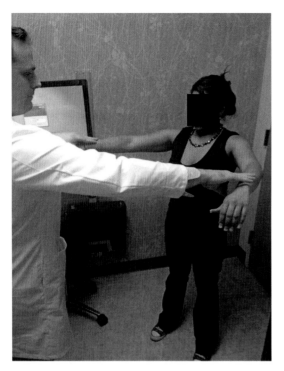

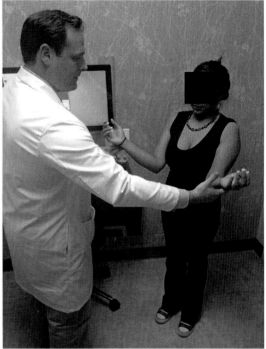

Fig. 2.1 The Jobe test, or "empty can test," is useful to evaluate for tears that involve the supraspinatus. The test is performed with the patient's shoulders flexed to 90° in the plane of the scapula and maximally internally rotated. The examiner then applies a downward force on the patients arm, and they are asked to resist. Weakness with this maneuver can indicate a tear in the supraspinatus tendon

Fig. 2.2 Resisted external rotation with the patient's arm at their side can indicate a tear that involves the infraspinatus when weakness is present

receives the injection, they should be examined again approximately 10 min later to allow the local anesthetic time to become effective. If a patient has adequate pain relief from the local anesthetic and is now able to elevate their arm above their head, then it can be surmised that pain inhibition is the true cause of their pseudoparalysis and not a biomechanical insufficiency. This information is useful in dictating future treatment options.

Targeted manual muscle testing of the rotator cuff should be performed. The Jobe test, or "empty can test," can be useful to test the integrity of the supraspinatus (Fig. 2.1). This test is performed with the shoulder abducted to horizontal, in the plane of the scapula, and internally rotated so the thumb is pointing to the floor. The examiner then applies a downward force on the arm and asks the patient to resist. The strength

can then be assessed. This test is only useful for patients who are able to elevate to horizontal against gravity. External rotation with the arm at the side can be useful in determining the strength of the infraspinatus (Fig. 2.2), while external rotation with the arm in 90° of abduction can be useful in isolating the teres minor. Subscapularis-specific testing such as the belly press (Fig. 2.3a), the bear hug (Fig. 2.3b), and the lift-off tests (Fig. 2.3c) can also be performed.

Lag signs are a useful adjunct to the physical examination and may be more sensitive and specific than manual muscle testing [8]. An external rotation lag can be evaluated with either the patient's arm at their side to evaluate for tears of the supraspinatus and infraspinatus (Fig. 2.4a, b) or in 90° of abduction to evaluate for teres minor insufficiency (Fig. 2.5a, b). Patients with massive rotator cuff tears often present with a large external rotation lag, as evidenced by a Hornblower's sign with functional activities [9]. This can often be ascertained upon initially greeting the patient

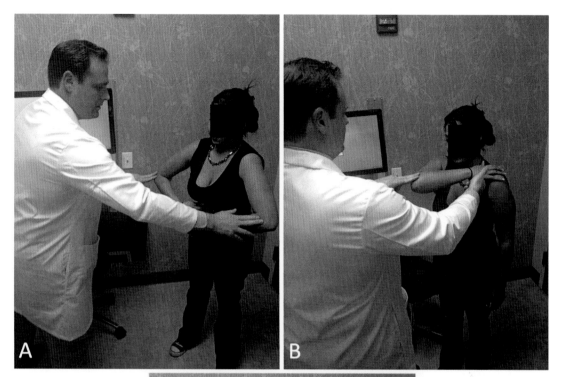

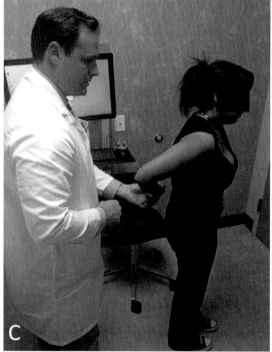

Fig. 2.3 The subscapularis can be tested through three commonly used tests. The belly press is the easiest for a patient with a painful shoulder to perform (**a**). This involves asking the patient to press their hands into their belly and move their elbows forward. A positive test is obtained with the patient's elbow drops back or is unable to be brought forward. The bear-hug test is also a useful test that many patients can easily perform (**b**). This involves having the patient place their hand on their opposite shoulder while elevating their elbow. The examiner then attempts to elevate the patient's hand off of their shoulder, and a positive test is obtained when this is easily accomplished. The lift-off test is typically very difficult to perform with patients with significant shoulder pain, or who lack enough internal rotation to put their arm behind their back (**c**). This test involves pulling the patient's hand away from their low back and asking them to hold it there. In a positive test, the hand falls back to the patient's back. Typically, all three tests can be used in conjunction with one another when examining a patient

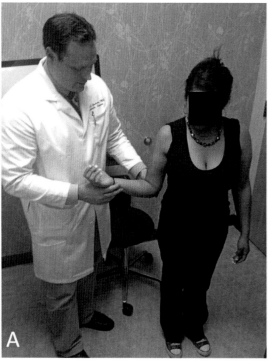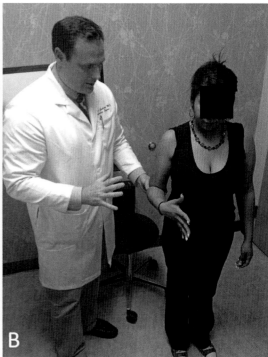

Fig. 2.4 An external rotation lag can be identified when the patient is unable to hold their arm in an externally rotated position. The examiner places the patient's arm in external rotation (**a**) and then asks them to hold it there. If the arm falls back in internal rotation, then the test is positive (**b**). This is indicative of a tear that involves the infraspinatus tendon

with a handshake. The Hornblower's sign is readily apparent if the patient's elbow goes away from their side as they attempt to elevate their shoulder. This can be a devastating functional problem since the shoulder external rotation with elevation is necessary to put the hand in a functional position to perform many activities of daily living, such as hair care.

Conclusion

The diagnosis of a massive rotator cuff tear can typically be made based on history and physical examination alone. In the history, it is most important to determine what the patient's chief complaint is whether it be pain, weakness, or a combination of both. In the physical examination, it is most important to determine whether or not the patient is able to elevate their arm. If they are not able to elevate their arm, it is important to determine whether or not they are unable to due to pain or biomechanical weakness. To delineate between the two, an injection with local anesthesia can be very effective at eliminating pain as a possible reason. If patients continue to have pseudoparalysis after an injection that achieves adequate pain relief, then it can be surmised that there is a biomechanical weakness. The history and physical examination does set forth a treatment algorithm for patients with massive rotator cuff tears. Comfort with these techniques comes with experience but is a crucial part in determining the adequate diagnosis and treatment options for these patients.

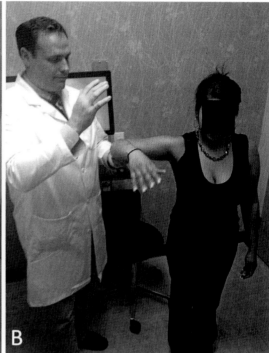

Fig. 2.5 A lag sign can be determined with the patient's shoulder in abduction. The examiner holds the patients shoulder in 90° of abduction and neutral rotation (hand facing the ceiling) (**a**). The patient is then asked to hold that position while the examiner lets go. If the arm goes into internal rotation, this is considered a positive test and is indicative of a tear that extends into the teres minor (**b**). Patients with external rotation lag with the arm in elevation are also said to have a Hornblower's sign. This can be a devastating functional problem since the shoulder external rotation with elevation is necessary to put the hand in a functional position to perform many activities of daily living, such as hair care

References

1. Boileau P, Baque F, Valerio L, Ahrens P, Chuinard C, Trojani C. Isolated arthroscopic biceps tenotomy or tenodesis improves symptoms in patients with massive irreparable rotator cuff tears. J Bone Joint Surg Am. 2007;89(4):747–57.
2. Fermont AJ, Wolterbeek N, Wessel RN, Baeyens JP, de Bie RA. Prognostic factors for successful recovery after arthroscopic rotator cuff repair: a systematic literature review. J Orthop Sports Phys Ther. 2014;44(3):153–63.
3. Clement ND, Hallett A, MacDonald D, Howie C, McBirnie J. Does diabetes affect outcome after arthroscopic repair of the rotator cuff? J Bone Joint Surg Br. 2010;92(8):1112–7.
4. Kukkonen J, Kauko T, Virolainen P, Aarimaa V. Smoking and operative treatment of rotator cuff tear. Scand J Med Sci Sports. 2014;24(2):400–3.
5. Titchener AG, White JJ, Hinchliffe SR, Tambe AA, Hubbard RB, Clark D. Comorbidities in rotator cuff disease: a case-control study. J Shoulder Elbow Surg. 2014;23(9):1282–8. doi:10.1016/j.jse.2013.12.019.
6. Harreld KL, Puskas BL, Frankle MA. Massive rotator cuff tears without arthropathy: when to consider reverse shoulder arthroplasty. Instr Course Lect. 2012;61:143–56.
7. Collin P, Matsumura N, Ladermann A, Denard PJ, Walch G. Relationship between massive chronic rotator cuff tear pattern and loss of active shoulder range of motion. J Shoulder Elbow Surg. 2014;23(8):1195–202. doi:10.1016/j.jse.2013.11.019.
8. Hertel R, Ballmer FT, Lombert SM, Gerber C. Lag signs in the diagnosis of rotator cuff rupture. J Shoulder Elbow Surg. 1996;5(4):307–13.
9. Walch G, Boulahia A, Calderone S, Robinson AH. The 'dropping' and 'hornblower's' signs in evaluation of rotator-cuff tears. J Bone Joint Surg Br. 1998;80(4):624–8.

Imaging of the Rotator Cuff

Gabrielle P. Konin

Pearls and Pitfalls

Pearls

- Not all massive rotator cuff tears are irreparable, and imaging findings that suggest irreparability include static superior migration of the humeral head with loss of the acromiohumeral interval and >50 % fatty infiltration of the muscles of the rotator cuff.
- On sonography, the absence of rotator cuff tissue over the humeral head filled with anechoic fluid or hypoechoic debris/granulation tissue is diagnostic of a full-thickness tear.
- As tendon retraction approaches the glenoid fossa, the more likely the tendon will be irreparable.
- An acute traumatic massive rotator cuff tear or avulsion will be hyperintense on MR imaging with surrounding soft tissue edema signal rather than the bland appearance typically seen with chronic tears. This is important to distinguish, as the repair of an inelastic poor quality tendon will have a poor postoperative prognosis.
- In cuff tear arthropathy, the glenoid fossa should be evaluated in both axial and coronal planes, which not only establishes the type of instability but also is important in preoperative assessment for glenoid baseplate fit. A glenoid vault measurement of <25 mm from glenoid face to the most medial cortex on the scapula using axial CT images suggests an inadequate bone stock for a glenoid baseplate – depending on the implant system used.

Pitfalls

- Granulation tissue can simulate cuff continuity on MR imaging as intermediate to high signal within the tendon gap.
- The infraspinatus, supraspinatus, and subscapularis muscles may appear falsely atrophic on sagittal images due to retraction of the muscle belly medial to the plane of imaging. Therefore, triangulation with coronal and axial oblique images to estimate the degree of retraction is helpful to properly assess the apparent atrophy.

G.P. Konin, MD (✉)
Department of Radiology and Imaging,
Hospital for Special Surgery,
535 E. 70th Street, New York, NY 10021, USA

Department of Radiology and Imaging, Weill Cornell Medical College, New York, NY, USA
e-mail: KoninG@hss.edu

L.V. Gulotta and E.V. Craig (eds.), *Massive Rotator Cuff Tears: Diagnosis and Management*,
DOI 10.1007/978-1-4899-7494-5_3, © Springer Science+Business Media New York 2015

- A nonfunctional deltoid, whether dehiscent or denervated, is a contraindication to the reverse TSA and can be readily assessed by MR imaging.
- Paralysis can mimic a rotator cuff tear clinically, and MR imaging aids in distinguishing the two. Paralysis due to subacute muscle denervation will appear as smooth homogeneous high signal throughout the muscle belly.

Introduction

Over the years, various imaging modalities have proved useful in the evaluation of the shoulder and its rotator cuff, each of which has its own advantages and disadvantages, with magnetic resonance (MR) imaging and ultrasound (US) used as the chief means to define rotator cuff pathology. A thorough understanding of the imaging characteristics and advantages of the various imaging modalities used to evaluate the rotator cuff, and in particular massive cuff tears, is essential for clinical decision making affording optimal treatment planning and information about prognosis.

MR imaging is the most commonly used imaging modality in the evaluation of rotator cuff pathology, with the capability of providing a comprehensive and detailed evaluation of the extent and configuration of rotator cuff tears [1]. It offers useful information regarding tendon/muscle quality, degree of tendon retraction, and possible cuff tear arthropathy and allows for an overall assessment of mechanical imbalances. Particular MR imaging findings relevant to massive rotator cuff tears will be addressed to help guide the complex decision-making process in management.

Sonography is a commonly used imaging modality in the evaluation of the rotator cuff and has the added advantage of dynamic scanning with provocative maneuvers that can reproduce symptoms [2]. Ultrasound can be an effective alternative for patients who are unable to undergo

MR imaging due to pacemakers and metallic implants – though dephasing artifact seen with metallic implants is less of an issue with current metal reduction techniques. Evaluation of complex tear patterns and the ability to grade fatty infiltration and assess intra-articular pathology remain limited with sonography [2].

CT can be used to assess the degree of atrophy and fatty infiltration of the cuff musculature and the osseous integrity of the glenoid for preoperative planning. Radiographs provide a simple and inexpensive means of assessing whether a massive cuff tear is likely and can demonstrate the presence of cuff tear arthropathy.

Massive Rotator Cuff Tear

Although there is no unified classification of massive rotator cuff tears by imaging, it is important to be aware of the various definitions in the literature. DeOrio and Cofield et al. classified rotator cuff tears by size in the anteroposterior dimension as either small (1 cm), medium (1–3 cm), large (3–5 cm), or massive (>5 cm) [3, 4] (Fig. 3.1), whereas Zumstein et al. provided an alternative definition, proposing that complete detachment of two or more tendons qualifies as a massive rotator cuff tear. Additional definitions have been formulated over the years by others [5–7]. Ultimately, relying on a solid understanding of the relevant imaging findings that lead to mechanical instability in combination with the clinical exam is most effective in driving management decisions and determining prognosis as restoration of mechanical balance is a primary goal.

As massive rotator cuff tears are not necessarily synonymous with irreparability, it is important to be aware of imaging signs suggesting when the rotator cuff is not likely to be reparable (see Pearls and Pitfalls). Markers that a rotator cuff tear is not amenable to anatomic repair include static superior migration of the humeral head, a narrowed or absent acromiohumeral interval, and >50 % fatty infiltration of the rotator cuff musculature [8].

On MRI, a full-thickness defect from the articular to the bursal surface should be identified with

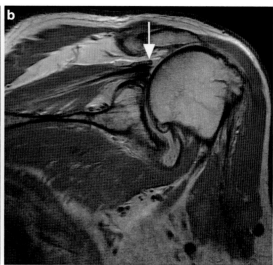

Fig. 3.1 Massive rotator cuff tear. (**a**) Sagittal oblique proton density-weighted MR image in an 83-year-old man demonstrates DeOrio and Cofield's classification of a chronic massive cuff tear spanning a distance of >5 cm (*double-headed arrow*). The defect in the infraspinatus and supraspinatus tendons extends from the articular surface to the bursal surface with loss of the acromio-humeral interval. (**b**) Coronal oblique proton density-weighted MR image demonstrates medial retraction of the supraspinatus tendon to the glenoid fossa (*arrow*) with mild fatty infiltration and mild to moderate decreased muscle bulk

reported sensitivities and specificities for the diagnosis of full-thickness tears on MRI ranging from 84 to 100 % and 93 to 99 %, respectively [1, 9]. It is important to be aware that a full-thickness fluid signal gap on fluid-sensitive and intermediate-weighted fast spin echo (FSE) MR sequences is not always demonstrated, and intermediate- to high-signal granulation tissue and/or synovial hypertrophy may fill the tear defect (see Pearls and Pitfalls). Once a full-thickness defect is confirmed and the tendon(s) identified, the anteroposterior dimension and the extent of tear propagation should be addressed. Attention should be paid to the integrity of the subscapularis and biceps long head tendons, as their status may alter prognosis with a torn subscapularis tendon potentially requiring an alternate surgical approach [10, 11].

Sonographic evaluation of massive rotator cuff tears should be performed in both the longitudinal axis (coronal) and short axis (transverse) imaging planes using a 9–15 MHz linear probe with the patient in the seated position. Massive cuff tears associated with rotator cuff tear arthropathy often provide a dilemma to the unsuspecting or inexperienced sonographer due to the altered anatomy afforded by the absent acromiohumeral interval. Furthermore, the inability of the patient to participate in maneuvers due to limited mobility and/or pain can make arriving at an imaging diagnosis difficult. Regardless of the limitations, the absence of rotator cuff tissue over the humeral head filled with anechoic fluid or hypoechoic debris/granulation tissue is diagnostic of a full-thickness tear (Fig. 3.2 and see Pearls and Pitfalls).

Tendon Retraction and Quality

The degree of tendon retraction plays a role in determining surgical reparability. The tendon is less likely to withstand the tensile load imparted on the repaired tendon when there is a greater degree of tendon retraction. This may tend toward a poor prognosis, and it is therefore important to assess at the time of MR imaging. As medial

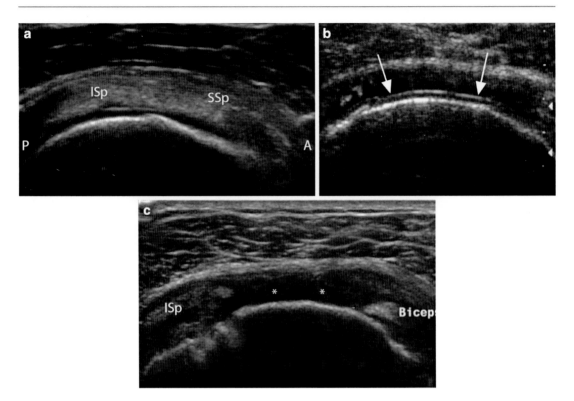

Fig. 3.2 Ultrasound of a massive rotator cuff tear. (**a**) Ultrasound image in the short axis demonstrates the normal supraspinatus and infraspinatus cuff tissue over the humeral head. (**b**) Short axis ultrasound image demonstrates complete full-thickness absence of the supraspinatus and infraspinatus tendons over the humeral head allowing for the cartilage to be seen (cartilage interface sign) (Ultrasound images courtesy of Dr. Gregory Saboeiro). (**c**) Ultrasound image in the short axis demonstrates absence of the supraspinatus tendon, which is filled with anechoic fluid (*asterisks*) and high-grade partial tearing of the infraspinatus (*ISp*)

retraction of the tendon approaches the glenoid fossa, the more likely the tendon will be irreparable [12] (Fig. 3.1 and see Pearls and Pitfalls), though be aware that the medial extent of tendon retraction as demonstrated at MR imaging may not represent true tendon retraction and may be mobile at arthroscopy. This typically depends on the chronicity of the tear as acute tears are more mobile than those that are chronic.

Although tendon tear shape is evaluated arthroscopically, the ability to detect tendon tear shapes decreases as the size of the tendon tear increases [13] with a limited role for MR imaging and less so for ultrasound. Massive contracted rotator cuff tears have been categorized into massive crescentic tears (wide anteroposterior dimension) and massive longitudinal tears (spared anterior cuff tissue at the rotator interval) [14].

Many cuff tears are reparable [14], and the ability to detect an acute traumatic massive cuff tear or avulsion rather than a chronic tear is important, as the acute tear will have good-quality elastic tendon stump and will not place undue tension on the tissue following repair. MR imaging can provide useful information about acuity and tendon quality given the degree or absence of soft tissue edema signal (Fig. 3.3). When the tear is chronic, it is important to evaluate the presence of degeneration characterized by fraying and irregularity and possible scarring, as the presumably poor-quality and/or inelastic tendon is unlikely to withstand suture anchoring and tension resulting in a poor postoperative prognosis (see Pearls and Pitfalls) [8].

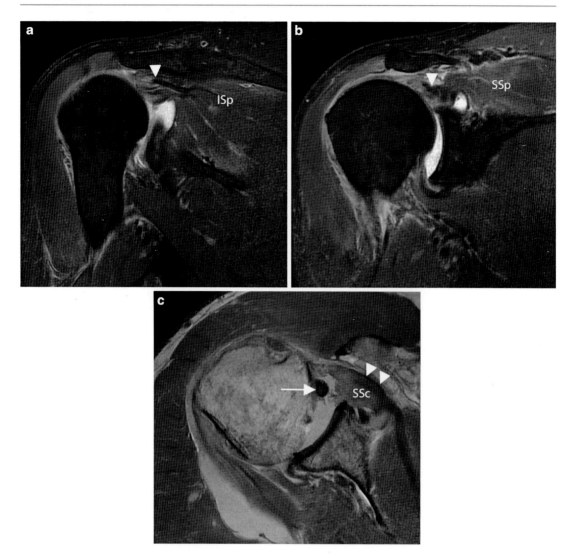

Fig. 3.3 Acute massive rotator cuff tear. (**a**, **b**) Coronal oblique fat-saturated T2- and (**c**) axial proton density-weighted MR images in a 55-year-old man status post a body-surfing injury reveals an acute traumatic avulsion of the infraspinatus (*ISp*), supraspinatus (*SSp*), and subscapularis (*SSc*) tendons (*arrowheads*) with edema signal extending medially within and around the muscle bellies. The biceps tendon has been destabilized and is medially dislocated to an intra-articular position (*arrow*)

Fatty Infiltration and Muscle Atrophy

Although degree of tendon retraction and tendon quality is important, it is the integrity of muscle quality that is integral in formulating a treatment plan. Fatty infiltration of the rotator cuff muscle belly has been established as a negative prognostic factor for reparability of the rotator cuff [12, 15–17].

It is therefore important to accurately assess the muscle quality using imaging, as surgical management and prognosis will be influenced by the status of muscle quality. The Goutallier classification of fatty infiltration, initially described using CT, is often applied in practice with MRI and US as they are currently the imaging modalities of choice in assessing the rotator cuff tendons. In clinical practice, modification of the Goutallier classification to a three-tiered staging system is

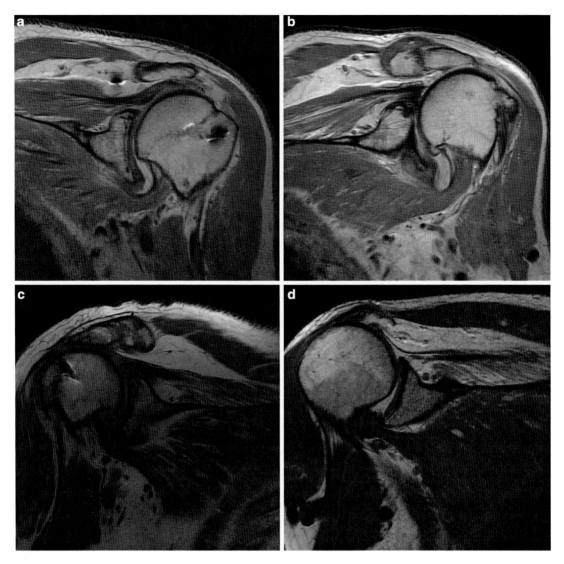

Fig. 3.4 Goutallier classification – applied to coronal oblique proton density MR images. (**a**) Mild (Goutallier stage 0 and stage 1) is defined as normal muscle without any or with minimal fatty streaks. (**b**) Moderate (Goutallier stage 2) is characterized by fatty infiltration, but there is more muscle than fat. (**c, d**) Severe (Goutallier stage 3 and stage 4), there is at least as much fatty infiltration as there is muscle

used to indicate the presence of fatty infiltration (Fig. 3.4): mild fatty infiltration (Goutallier stage 0 and stage 1) indicates normal muscle without or with minimal fatty streaks; moderate fatty infiltration (Goutallier stage 2) is characterized by fatty infiltration, but more muscle than fat; and severe fatty infiltration (Goutallier stage 3 and stage 4) demonstrates at least as much fatty infiltration as there is muscle. Warner et al. evaluated the degree of fatty infiltration in massive rotator cuff tears of the same size and found correlation between the degree of fatty infiltration on MRI and overall biomechanics and function [11, 15].

Ultrasound can be used to evaluate the degree of muscle atrophy and fatty infiltration with good correlation with MR imaging [18] – nevertheless, this remains challenging and is user dependent. Fatty infiltration will be seen as effacement of the normal pennate pattern of the muscle and increased hyperechogenicity (Fig. 3.5). It is often helpful to

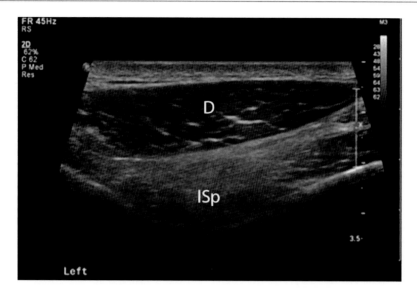

Fig. 3.5 Ultrasound of fatty infiltration. Short axis ultrasound image shows hyperechogenicity of the infraspinatus (*ISp*) muscle belly as compared to the normal appearance of the overlying deltoid muscle (*D*), which is indicative of fatty infiltration (Ultrasound image courtesy of Dr. Gregory Saboeiro)

compare the degree of echogenicity with the overlying deltoid or trapezius muscles and the adjacent teres minor muscle when they are normal.

Methods to assess supraspinatus muscle atrophy include the scapular occupation ratio and the "tangent sign." It is important to recognize the difference between loss of muscle bulk and true fatty infiltration. Muscle atrophy has the potential to be reversible if fatty infiltration is not present. Zanetti and coworkers described the "tangent sign" to assess muscle atrophy in the sagittal oblique plane on MRI at the medial coracoid process [19] (Fig. 3.6). The normal supraspinatus muscle belly should cross superior to a line across the superior borders of the scapular spine and the superior margin of the coracoid process. With an atrophic muscle belly, the muscle will lie inferior to the line.

Thomazeau described the occupation ratio, which is evaluated in the same imaging plane and utilizing the same osseous landmarks [12]. It is defined as the ratio of the cross-sectional area of the supraspinatus muscle to the area of the supraspinatus fossa, with a ratio of less than 50 % indicative of muscle atrophy (Fig. 3.7). This method was shown to correlate supraspinatus atrophy with the extent of tendon tear and was associated with postoperative tear recurrence. Both methods have been shown to correlate with strength and mobil-

ity. When evaluating the cross-sectional area of the supraspinatus and other cuff tendons, it is important to be aware of the degree of tendon retraction as this can result in an overestimation of muscle atrophy if the torn tendon has retracted far medially (see Pearls and Pitfalls). Cross-referencing with the coronal and axial planes and awareness of the marbling due to fatty infiltration should help one avoid this imaging pitfall (Fig. 3.8). Cross-sectional areas of the infraspinatus, teres minor, and subscapularis muscles have also been correlated with chronicity of rotator cuff tears, with the subscapularis muscle atrophy being associated with poorer surgical outcomes [11, 19].

It is important to recognize subacute muscle denervation involving one or more muscle groups of the shoulder girdle, such as seen with Parsonage-Turner syndrome (inflammation of the brachial plexus). Although, subacute denervation is rare, it can mimic the clinical presentation of pseudoparalysis seen with a massive rotator cuff tear (see Pearls and Pitfalls). Subacute muscle denervation causes diffuse homogenous edema signal confined to the involved muscle and is usually evident on MR imaging 2–4 weeks after denervation has occurred [20] (Fig. 3.9). This can be distinguished from acute muscle injury, as muscle injury characteristically manifests as a feathery edema pattern

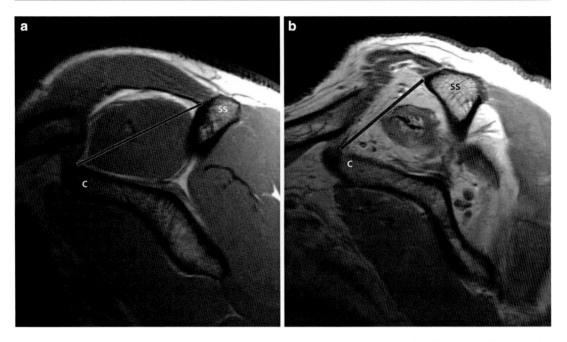

Fig. 3.6 Tangent sign. (**a**) Sagittal oblique proton density-weighted MR image shows the muscle belly of the normal supraspinatus muscle crossing a tangent (*line*) drawn between the superior borders of the scapular spine

(*ss*) and the superior margin of the coracoid process (*c*). (**b**) Sagittal proton density-weighted MR image demonstrates atrophy of the supraspinatus muscle, which now lies below the tangent (*line*)

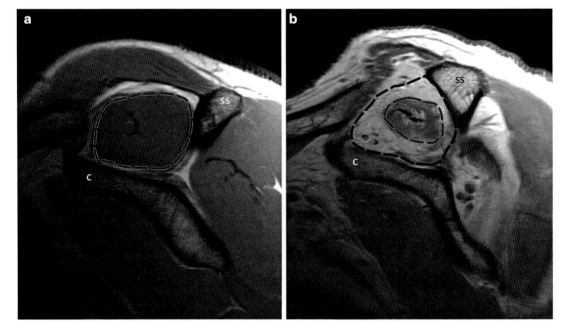

Fig. 3.7 Occupation ratio. (**a**) Sagittal oblique proton density-weighted MR image shows a normal occupation ratio, representing the ratio between the cross-sectional area of the belly of the supraspinatus muscle (*red-dashed line*) and that of the scapular fossa (*red-dashed line*). (**b**)

Sagittal oblique proton density-weighted MR image demonstrates volume loss in the supraspinatus muscle belly (*red-dashed line*) with a smaller cross-sectional area compared to that of the scapular fossa (*black-dashed line*). *c* coracoid process, *ss* scapular spine

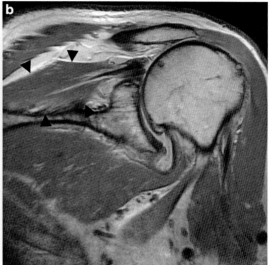

Fig. 3.8 Pitfall in estimation of muscle atrophy. (**a**) Sagittal oblique proton density-weighted MR image shows both an abnormal tangent sign and occupation ratio. However, it is important to not overestimate the degree of atrophy as the supraspinatus tendon may be retracted medially. (**b**) Coronal oblique proton density-weighted MR image demonstrates medial retraction of the muscle belly (*arrowheads*), which is not as atrophic as might be expected based on the tangent sign/occupation ratio determined on sagittal oblique imaging alone

and often has adjacent edema signal within the soft tissues. Acute, traumatic edema is typically seen within hours to days after injury. If innervation is restored, the MR imaging findings will return to normal. If not restored, a chronic irreversible denervation will ensue characterized by fatty infiltration. If denervation is suspected, correlation with electromyographic findings and a careful search for upper extremity peripheral nerve compression by a mass lesion should be performed. Parsonage-Turner syndrome is usually self-limited with a return to full recovery as the rule.

Long Head of the Biceps Tendon

The condition of the long head of the biceps tendon may be evaluated preoperatively by either MRI or ultrasound. In particular, it is important to note its position as to whether it is centered, subluxed, dislocated, or frankly ruptured. Often with massive rotator cuff tears, the long head of the biceps tendon is ruptured with its intracapsular course no longer visualized on MR imaging. High-grade or full-thickness subscapularis tendon tears should direct one's attention to the long

head of the biceps for subluxation or dislocation (Fig. 3.3). Ultrasound plays a role in evaluating the long head of the biceps tendon; however, the proximal intracapsular course of the tendon is not amenable to sonographic visualization.

Rotator Cuff Tear Arthropathy

A massive rotator cuff tear is required for rotator cuff tear arthropathy (CTA), but not everyone with massive rotator cuff tears develops CTA. The exact etiology of cuff arthropathy, though unknown, is likely multifactorial and can be associated with inflammatory and crystalline arthropathies [10, 21, 22]. Imaging plays an important role in establishing the diagnosis of CTA and provides important information to guide management. When evaluating for CTA on imaging, one should be aware of the transverse and/or coronal force coupling deficiencies that exist. These coupling deficiencies result in failure to constrain and center the humeral head within the glenoid resulting in abnormal physical stresses secondarily imparted to the humeral head. This can ultimately lead to the gradual anterosuperior migration and wear on

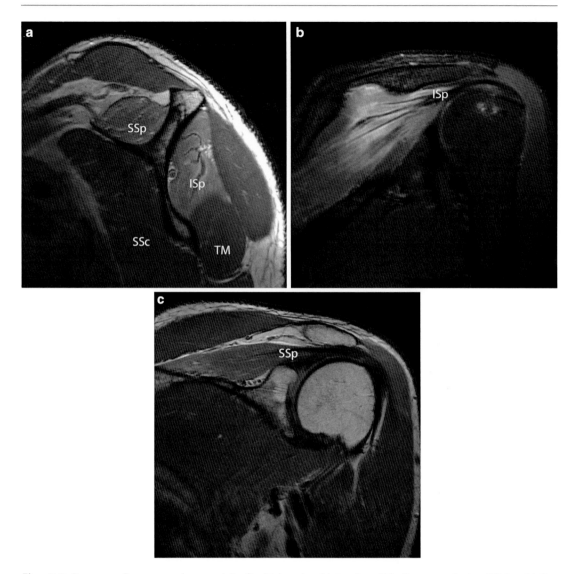

Fig. 3.9 Parsonage-Turner syndrome. (**a**) Sagittal oblique proton density-, (**b**) coronal oblique fat-saturated T2-, and (**c**) coronal oblique proton density-weighted MR images show diffuse homogeneous abnormal high signal intensity within the supraspinatus (*SSp*) and infraspinatus (*ISp*) muscle bellies without rotator cuff tear. The subscapularis muscle (*SSc*) and teres minor muscle (*TM*) are normal

the glenoid. The Neer definition of CTA includes glenohumeral arthrosis, superior migration of the humeral head with collapse of the proximal humeral articular surface, and erosion with eventual acetabularization of the acromion [8, 22].

Radiographs with anteroposterior (AP) and axillary views are often sufficient for the diagnosis of cuff tear arthropathy. They are used to reveal the presence of static superior migration of the humeral head with subacromial remodeling and glenohumeral wear at various stages, as initially classified by Hamada et al. in 1990 [23]. The acromiohumeral interval should be no less than 7 mm as measured on the neutral AP or Grashey view. Grade 1 rotator cuff tear arthrosis indicates an acromiohumeral interval ≥6 mm; grade 2 is determined by acromiohumeral interval ≤5 mm; grade 3 is ≤5 mm with acetabularization; grade 4A involves glenohumeral arthrosis without acetabularization and grade 4B is glenohumeral arthrosis with acetabularization; and grade 5 indicates articular surface erosive wear and/or collapse of the humeral head (Fig. 3.10).

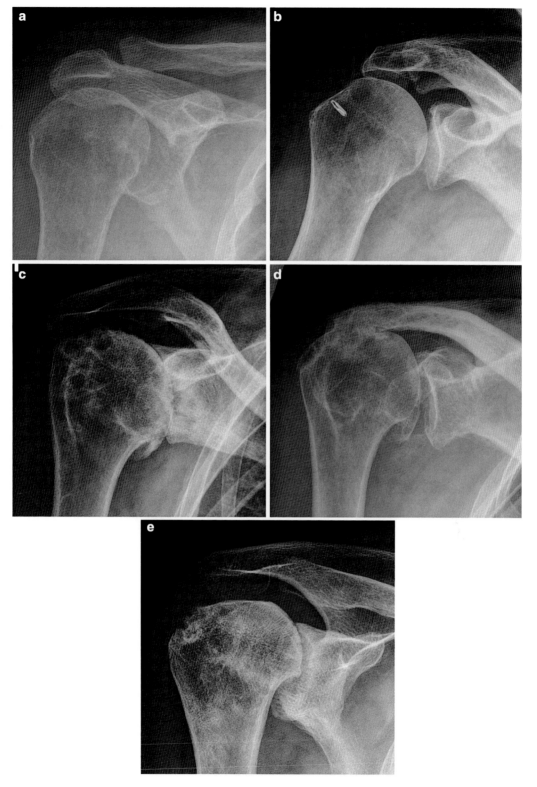

Fig. 3.10 Hamada classification. AP neutral radiographs demonstrate (**a**) Hamada grade 2 CTA with an acromiohumeral interval (AHI) ≤5 mm, (**b**) Hamada grade 3 CTA with an acromiohumeral interval ≤5 mm and acetabularization of the acromion, (**c**) Hamada grade 4A CTA with glenohumeral arthrosis but no acetabularization, (**d**) Hamada grade 4B CTA with glenohumeral arthrosis and acetabularization, and (**e**) Hamada grade 5 with glenohumeral arthrosis and humeral articular surface collapse

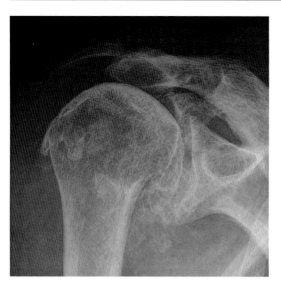

Fig. 3.11 Stress fracture of the acromion. AP radiograph in external rotation shows CTA in a 78-year-old woman with acetabularization of the acromion and a fracture of the acromion process due to the high contact forces from the superiorly subluxed humeral head

Progressive osseous erosion of the undersurface of the acromion can progress to acromial stress reactions/fractures (Fig. 3.11) [10]. Radiographs can detect disuse osteopenia of the acromion and proximal humerus as the patient attempts to protect the shoulder.

CT is typically the preferred imaging modality for presurgical planning as it provides excellent osseous visualization. With anterior superior migration of the humeral head, CT can demonstrate wear of both the humeral and glenoid articular surfaces and with more advanced anterosuperior escape, the coracoid process. While standard osteoarthritis of the shoulder commonly results in wear on the posterior aspect of the glenoid, CTA typically causes anterosuperior glenoid wear due to the superior migration of the humeral head. Walch et al. and Sirveaux et al. have classified glenoid morphology in the axial and coronal planes, respectively [24, 25]. In the system described by Sirveaux and associates, type E0 represents no glenoid wear, type E1 describes central glenoid wear, type E2 characterizes superior glenoid wear with superior biconcavity, and type E3 indicates severe supe-

rior glenoid wear extending inferiorly and reorienting the glenoid articular surface to a superiorly tilted position. These latter stages that involve superior glenoid wear are important to recognize since bone grafting may be necessary to accurately place the glenoid component of a reverse shoulder arthroplasty in the proper neutral or inferiorly tilted position (Fig. 3.12).

The classification system described by Walch and colleagues in the axial plane for primary osteoarthrosis describes a type A1 glenoid with minor osseous erosion as a result of concentric loading, type A2 glenoid that is due to concentric loading with excessive central wear, type B1 glenoid that is characterized by eccentric loading causing posterior subluxation of the humeral head with mild posterior joint wear, type B2 glenoid that is defined by eccentric loading with posterior subluxation of the humeral head yielding excessive posterior glenoid wear and biconcavity, and type C glenoid as frankly dysplastic with severe posterior glenoid wear (Fig. 3.13). Axial CT and MR images provide evaluation of the glenoid vault. At least 25 mm of the bone from the glenoid face to the most medial cortex of the scapula is necessary to provide adequate implantation of the baseplate, though this varies for different implant systems (Fig. 3.14 and see Pearls and Pitfalls) [26]. The wear patterns typically seen in osteoarthritis are important to recognize as the indications for reverse shoulder arthroplasty continue to expand.

Though MR imaging may not be necessary in diagnosing a massive cuff tear or cuff tear arthropathy, it can aid in the assessment of cuff reparability and centering of the humeral head and can ultimately assist in determining what type of arthroplasty is indicated: total shoulder arthroplasty (TSA), if the cuff is reparable, versus a hemiarthroplasty or reverse TSA, if the cuff is irreparable. Contraindications to the popularized reverse TSA are an inadequate glenoid vault as well as a nonfunctional deltoid, both of which can be readily assessed on MR imaging (Figs. 3.15 and 3.16). Assessment of deltoid dysfunction is important, as the reverse TSA depends

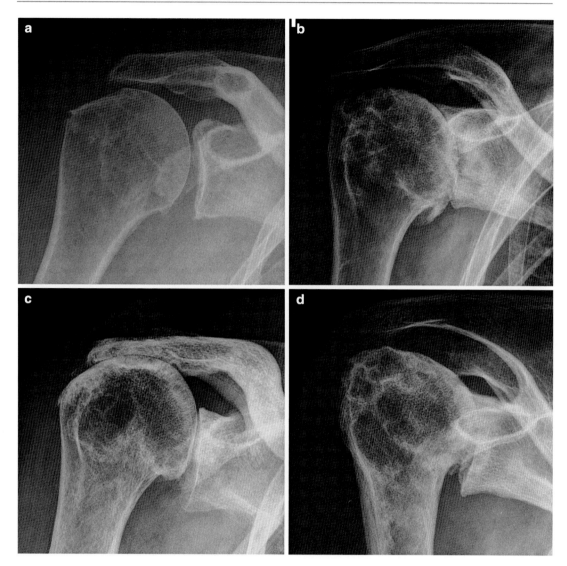

Fig. 3.12 Sirveaux classification. AP neutral radiographs demonstrate (**a**) type E0 represents no glenoid wear, (**b**) type E1 characterizes central glenoid wear, (**c**) type E2 indicates superior glenoid wear with superior biconcavity, and (**d**) type E3 represents severe superior glenoid wear extending inferiorly with redirection of the glenoid surface to a superiorly tilted orientation

on the deltoid muscle to act as a primary lever arm (see Pearls and Pitfalls). An incompetent CA ligament is not a contraindication for reverse TSA as it is in the other types of prostheses. In addition, the status of the articular cartilage can be readily assessed on MRI – classically, with loss of anterosuperior glenoid articular cartilage and eventual glenohumeral osseous remodeling due to the load imparted by the anterosuperior humeral head escape.

Ultrasound plays a limited role in evaluation of cuff tear arthropathy and can ultimately prove confusing in inexperienced hands given the superior migration of the humeral head and its

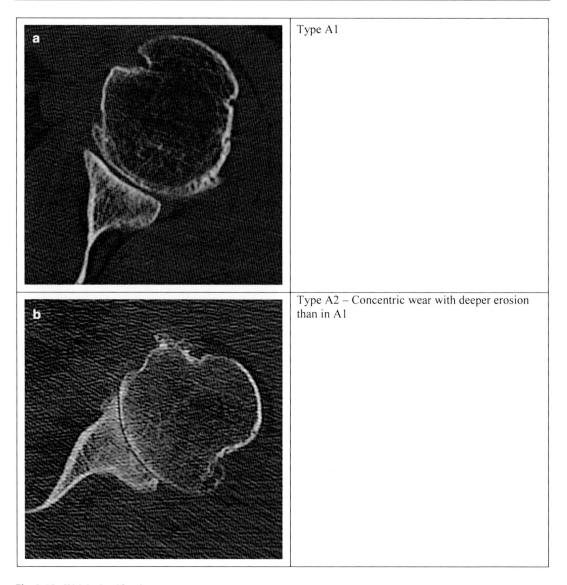

Type A1

Type A2 – Concentric wear with deeper erosion than in A1

Fig. 3.13 Walch classification

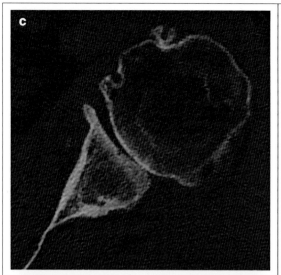

Type B1 – Posterior wear resulting in narrowing of the joint space, subchondral sclerosis, and osteophytes

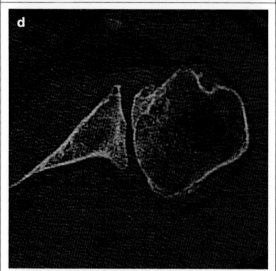

Type B2 – Posterior wear yielding a biconcave shape

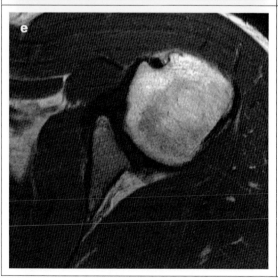

Type C – Dysplastic glenoid retroversion of more than 25 degrees and posterior subluxation of the humerus

Fig. 3.13 (continued)

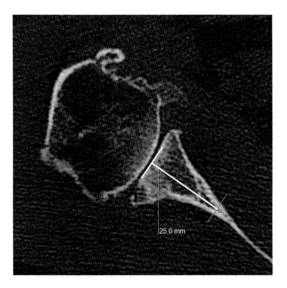

Fig. 3.14 Glenoid vault measurement. Axial CT image demonstrates the method for measuring the glenoid vault, which is adequate in this patient, measuring 25 mm

close apposition with the acromion. If there is concern whether synovitis and/or bursitis is associated with an inflammatory arthropathy or infection, guided aspiration may be performed, typically yielding a large amount of aseptic blood-tinged fluid (Fig. 3.17). Ultrasound-guided injections may also serve as an important tool in the treatment of patients with CTA.

Postoperative Rotator Cuff

Imaging evaluation of the postoperative cuff can be challenging. In order to achieve optimal evaluation, the radiologist and the orthopedic surgeon need to have a working relationship such that the radiologist is familiar with the surgical techniques employed by their referring clinician. In the postoperative evaluation of a repaired

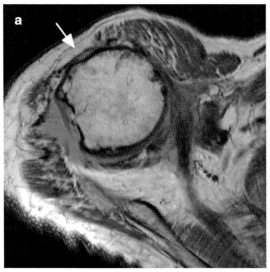

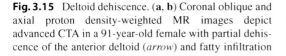

Fig. 3.15 Deltoid dehiscence. (**a, b**) Coronal oblique and axial proton density-weighted MR images depict advanced CTA in a 91-year-old female with partial dehiscence of the anterior deltoid (*arrow*) and fatty infiltration

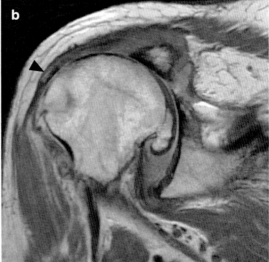

of the remaining deltoid muscle. On the coronal image, the deltoid dehiscence is associated with a small osseous avulsion fragment (*arrowhead*). Note the slightly superiorly directed glenoid – Sirveaux type E3

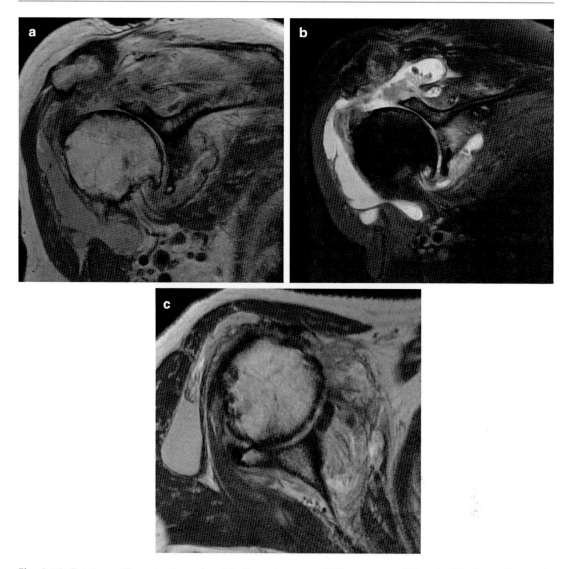

Fig. 3.16 Rotator cuff tear arthropathy. (**a**) Coronal oblique proton density-, (**b**) coronal oblique fat-saturated T2-, and (**c**) axial proton density-weighted MR images show advanced CTA with remodeling of the glenoid in the coronal (Sirveaux type E1) and axial planes (Walch A2) with a glenoid vault measurement of 15 mm and fragmentation anteriorly, rendering the glenoid vault potentially insufficient for a standard baseplate

massive cuff tear, the surgeon may choose a non-anatomical repair with partial repair leaving a gap in the cuff that should not be mistaken for a recurrent tear. Furthermore, the tendon-bone junction may no longer be anatomic and the repaired tendon may be medialized simulating a tear at the footprint. Massive recurrent tears are typically indisputable by both sonographic and MR imaging (Fig. 3.18); however, the exact extent of the re-tear may, at times, may be in question. Surgical techniques employed for irreparable cuff tears may require salvage treatment with various tendon transfers and other less commonly used treatment regimens, such as the utilization of scaffolds that may pose imaging challenges. Dynamic sonographic interrogation to visualize the continuity of the tendon with extensive postsurgical changes can prove useful when the diagnosis of a re-tear is in question. Suture anchors may result in focal acoustic

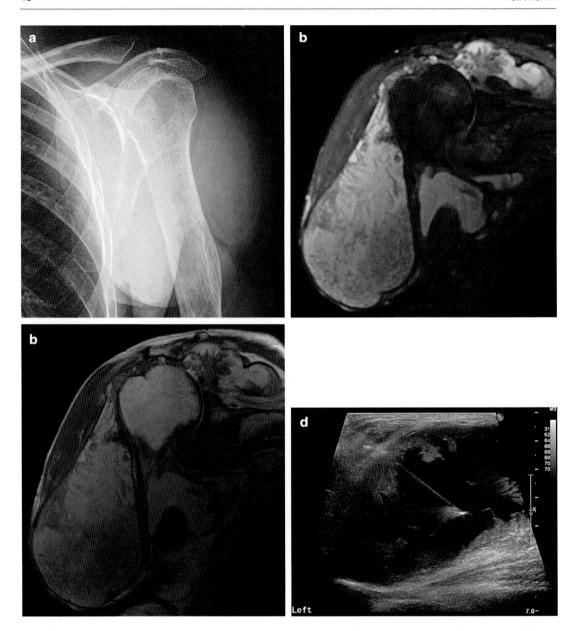

Fig. 3.17 Rheumatoid arthritis and CTA. (**a**) AP neutral radiograph demonstrates CTA in a 63-year-old woman with long-standing rheumatoid arthritis shows advanced CTA with a large soft tissue mass. (**b, c**) Coronal oblique proton density- and fat-saturated T2-weighted MR images demonstrate a striking inflammatory synovitis decom- pressing into the subacromial subdeltoid space and form- ing a geyser sign with decompression through an incompetent AC joint. (**d**) Ultrasound-guided aspiration yielded a substantial amount of blood-tinged synovial fluid. Note the prominent synovial fronds on sonography

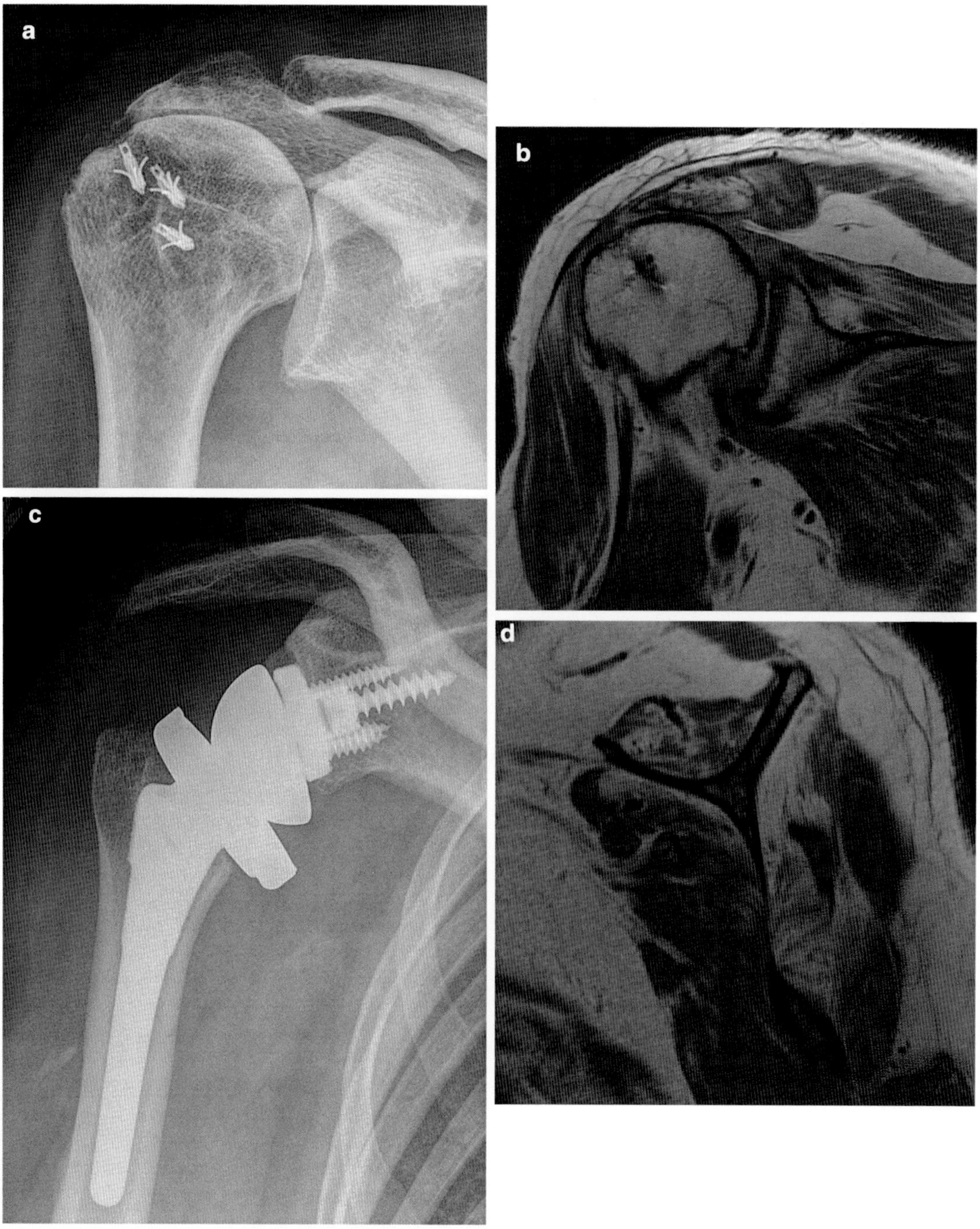

Fig. 3.18 Supraspinatus and infraspinatus re-tear. (**a**) AP external rotation radiograph in a 72-year-old man status post rotator cuff repair demonstrates superior escape of the humeral head due to recurrent cuff tear, resulting in acetabularization of the acromion and mild glenohumeral osteoarthrosis (Hamada Grade 4B). (**b**) Coronal oblique proton density-, (**c**) coronal oblique fat-saturated T2-, and (**d**) sagittal oblique proton density-weighted images demonstrate advanced CTA with moderate supraspinatus and severe infraspinatus fatty infiltration with preservation of the subscapularis and deltoid muscle. (**e**) The patient underwent a reverse total shoulder arthroplasty

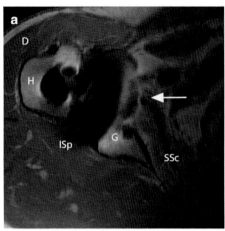

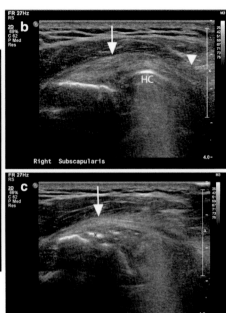

Fig. 3.19 Subscapularis tear with pectoralis transfer. (**a**) Axial oblique proton density MR image demonstrates a total shoulder arthroplasty in a 65-year-old man with subscapularis (*SSC*) tendon dehiscence and medial retraction (*arrow*) to the glenoid fossa. Mild fatty infiltration can be seen in the subscapularis muscle. The supraspinatus (*SSP*) and infraspinatus (*ISP*) tendons were shown to be intact and the deltoid (*D*) was not dehiscent. (**b, c**) The patient eventually underwent a pectoralis major tendon transfer and later developed acute pain in which dynamic sonographic imaging in the long axis determined the pectoralis transfer (*arrows*) to be intact, *HC* humeral component, *asterisk* surgical sutures, *arrowhead* glenohumeral joint line

shadowing, which should not be mistaken for a tear. Following arthroplasty, both ultrasound and MR imaging utilizing metallic reduction software may be used to evaluate the integrity of the cuff (Fig. 3.19).

Conclusion

Imaging is a critical component in the evaluation of massive rotator cuff tears. MR remains the chief imaging modality, though plain radiographs, ultrasound, and CT can also provide valuable information. Factors such as humeral head elevation, tendon retraction, and fatty infiltration of the muscle belly are all poor prognostic imaging findings in terms of whether a tear is reparable or not.

References

1. Iannotti JP, Zlatkin MB, Esterhai JL, Kressel HY, Dalinka MK, Spindler KP. Magnetic resonance imaging of the shoulder. Sensitivity, specificity, and predictive value. J Bone Joint Surg Am. 1991;73(1):17–29.
2. Teefey SA, Rubin DA, Middleton WD, Hildebolt CF, Leibold RA, Yamaguchi K. Detection and quantification of rotator cuff tears. Comparison of ultrasonographic, magnetic resonance imaging, and arthroscopic findings in seventy-one consecutive cases. J Bone Joint Surg Am. 2004;86-A(4):708–16.
3. Cofield RH, Parvizi J, Hoffmeyer PJ, Lanzer WL, Ilstrup DM, Rowland CM. Surgical repair of chronic rotator cuff tears. A prospective long-term study. J Bone Joint Surg Am. 2001;83-A(1):71–7. PubMed PMID: 11205861.
4. DeOrio JK, Cofield RH. Results of a second attempt at surgical repair of a failed initial rotator-cuff repair. J Bone Joint Surg Am. 1984;66(4):563–7. PubMed PMID: 6707035.

5. Burkhart SS, Barth JR, Richards DP, Zlatkin MB, Larsen M. Arthroscopic repair of massive rotator cuff tears with stage 3 and 4 fatty degeneration. Arthroscopy. 2007;23(4):347–54. PubMed PMID: 17418325.

6. Tauro JC. Stiffness and rotator cuff tears: incidence, arthroscopic findings, and treatment results. Arthroscopy. 2006;22(6):581–6. PubMed PMID: 16762694.

7. Zumstein MA, Jost B, Hempel J, Hodler J, Gerber C. The clinical and structural long-term results of open repair of massive tears of the rotator cuff. J Bone Joint Surg Am. 2008;90(11):2423–31. doi:10.2106/JBJS.G.00677. PubMed PMID: 18978411.

8. Bedi A, Dines J, Warren RF, Dines DM. Massive tears of the rotator cuff. J Bone Joint Surg Am. 2010; 92(9):1894–908. doi:10.2106/JBJS.I.01531. Review. PubMed PMID: 20686065.

9. Quinn SF, Sheley RC, Demlow TA, Szumowski J. Rotator cuff tendon tears: evaluation with fat-suppressed MR imaging with arthroscopic correlation in 100 patients. Radiology. 1995;195(2):497–500. PubMed PMID: 7724773.

10. Feeley BT, Gallo RA, Craig EV. Cuff tear arthropathy: current trends in diagnosis and surgical management. J Shoulder Elbow Surg. 2009;18(3):484–94. doi:10.1016/j.jse.2008.11.003. Epub 2009 Feb 8. Review. PubMed PMID: 19208484.

11. Warner JJ, Higgins L, Parsons 4th IM, Dowdy P. Diagnosis and treatment of anterosuperior rotator cuff tears. J Shoulder Elbow Surg. 2001;10(1):37–46. PubMed PMID: 11182734.

12. Thomazeau H, Boukobza E, Morcet N, Chaperon J, Langlais F. Prediction of rotator cuff repair results by magnetic resonance imaging. Clin Orthop Relat Res. 1997;344:275–83. PubMed PMID: 9372778.

13. Gartsman GM, Hammerman SM. Full-thickness tears: arthroscopic repair. Orthop Clin North Am. 1997;28(1):83–98. PubMed PMID: 9024434.

14. Lo IK, Burkhart SS. Arthroscopic repair of massive, contracted, immobile rotator cuff tears using single and double interval slides: technique and preliminary results. Arthroscopy. 2004;20(1):22–33. PubMed PMID: 14716275.

15. Burkhart SS. Arthroscopic treatment of massive rotator cuff tears. Clinical results and biomechanical rationale. Clin Orthop Relat Res. 1991;267:45–56. PubMed PMID: 2044292.

16. Goutallier D, Postel JM, Zilber S, Van Driessche S. Shoulder surgery: from cuff repair to joint replacement. An update. Joint Bone Spine. 2003;70(6):422–32. PubMed PMID: 14667550.

17. Goutallier D, Postel JM, Bernageau J, Lavau L, Voisin MC. Fatty muscle degeneration in cuff ruptures. Pre- and postoperative evaluation by CT scan. Clin Orthop Relat Res. 1994;304:78–83. PubMed PMID: 8020238.

18. Khoury V, Cardinal E, Brassard P. Atrophy and fatty infiltration of the supraspinatus muscle: sonography versus MRI. AJR Am J Roentgenol. 2008;190(4):1105–11. doi:10.2214/AJR.07.2835. PubMed PMID: 18356462.

19. Zanetti M, Gerber C, Hodler J. Quantitative assessment of the muscles of the rotator cuff with magnetic resonance imaging. Invest Radiol. 1998;33(3):163–70. PubMed PMID: 9525755.

20. May DA, Disler DG, Jones EA, Balkissoon AA, Manaster BJ. Abnormal signal intensity in skeletal muscle at MR imaging: patterns, pearls, and pitfalls. Radiographics. 2000;20 Spec No:S295–315. Review. PubMed PMID: 11046180.

21. Ecklund KJ, Lee TQ, Tibone J, Gupta R. Rotator cuff tear arthropathy. J Am Acad Orthop Surg. 2007;15(6):340–9. Review. PubMed PMID: 17548883.

22. Jensen KL, Williams Jr GR, Russell IJ, Rockwood Jr CA. Rotator cuff tear arthropathy. J Bone Joint Surg Am. 1999;81(9):1312–24. Review. PubMed PMID: 10505528.

23. Hamada K, Fukuda H, Mikasa M, Kobayashi Y. Roentgenographic findings in massive rotator cuff tears. A long-term observation. Clin Orthop Relat Res. 1990;254:92–6. PubMed PMID: 2323152.

24. Sirveaux F, Favard L, Oudet D, Huquet D, Walch G, Molé D. Grammont inverted total shoulder arthroplasty in the treatment of glenohumeral osteoarthritis with massive rupture of the cuff. Results of a multicentre study of 80 shoulders. J Bone Joint Surg Br. 2004;86(3):388–95.

25. Walch G, Badet R, Boulahia A, Khoury A. Morphologic study of the glenoid in primary glenohumeral osteoarthritis. J Arthroplasty. 1999;14(6):756–60. PubMed PMID: 10512449.

26. Frankle M, Siegal S, Pupello D, Saleem A, Mighell M, Vasey M. The Reverse Shoulder Prosthesis for glenohumeral arthritis associated with severe rotator cuff deficiency. A minimum two-year follow-up study of sixty patients. J Bone Joint Surg Am. 2005;87(8):1697–705. PubMed PMID: 16085607.

Nonoperative Management: Natural History, Medications, and Injections

4

Bashar Alolabi and Eric T. Ricchetti

Pearls and Pitfalls of Steroid Injections

Pearls
- In massive rotator cuff tears, a subacromial steroid injection also becomes an intra-articular glenohumeral injection
- Injections can be performed from an anterior, posterior, or lateral approach based on clinician preference, bony anatomy, and patient body habitus
- An anterior injection may provide easier access to the glenohumeral joint in a larger patient, as the soft tissue distance the needle must traverse is less because of the deltopectoral interval and rotator interval
- In a patient with superior migration of the humeral head and a decreased acromiohumeral interval, an anterior or posterior injection approach may be preferred

Pitfalls
- Avoid injecting when significant resistance is felt, as this may be a sign of intramuscular or intratendinous needle position and potential risk of muscle or tendon rupture
- Skin depigmentation at the injection site can occur, particularly in darker-skinned individuals
- Elevation of blood sugar levels may occur in diabetic patients
- Avoid too frequent or an excessive number of injections. Excessive injections can play a role in the development of deltoid ruptures or may eventually weaken the remaining rotator cuff tissue

Background

Rotator cuff tears are common and increase in frequency with advancing age [1]. The prevalence of rotator cuff tears averages 20 %, increasing to over 50 % in people over 80 years old [2, 3]. The most susceptible tendon to rupture is that of the supraspinatus muscle [4–6]. Although there is some controversy regarding the definition of a massive rotator cuff tear, many authors define a tear involving at least two tendons and/or measuring more than 5 cm in the anteroposterior width as

B. Alolabi, MD, FRCSC
Department of Orthopaedic Surgery, Sunnybrook Health Sciences Centre, 2501-3303 Don Mills Rd, Toronto, ON M2J 4T6, USA
e-mail: balolabi@gmail.com

E.T. Ricchetti, MD (✉)
Department of Orthopaedic Surgery, The Cleveland Clinic, Mail Code A40, 9500 Euclid Ave, Cleveland, OH, USA
e-mail: eric.ricchetti@gmail.com

massive [7, 8]. Massive tears are usually chronic in nature and rarely due to an acute injury. As such, they are generally associated with myotendinous retraction [1, 9, 10], loss of musculotendinous elasticity [11], fatty infiltration and muscle atrophy [12], and eventual development of static superior subluxation of the humeral head with associated degenerative changes [1, 13–16].

Even though patients with rotator cuff tears are often asymptomatic [17, 18], approximately 34.6 % of subjects with rotator cuff tears develop pain and shoulder disability [1, 6], including weakness with the arm away from the body [19]. Massive tears are more commonly associated with weakness [20] and often painful disability [8].

Massive tears are classified as anterosuperior or posterosuperior, each with unique incidence, clinical presentation, examination findings, and prognosis [21]. Anterosuperior tears involve a complete tear of the supraspinatus and the subscapularis tendons. These tears may be associated with instability or rupture of the long head of the biceps tendon. If the coracoacromial arch is violated, these anterosuperior tears may also result in superior escape of the humeral head and the development of pseudoparalysis [21]. Posterosuperior tears involve the supraspinatus and infraspinatus tendons and lead to the disruption of the balance of forces at the shoulder [22], resulting in superior and anterosuperior migration of the humeral head and subsequently, abnormal loading of the glenoid [23]. This abnormal mechanical loading has been implicated as the primary initiating mechanism of rotator cuff tear arthropathy [24–26]. These changes lead to altered mechanics not only of the glenohumeral joint but also of the shoulder and periscapular musculature and result in significant pain and dysfunction, including the potential development of pseudoparalysis [23].

The management of massive rotator cuff tears is complex due to the many involved variables, such as patient age, quality of the ruptured rotator cuff tissue, chronicity of the tear, patient activity level, degree of muscle atrophy and fatty infiltration, presence of arthritis, and other patient medical comorbidities. The management of these types of tears is typically focused on pain reduction and functional improvement [23]. Whereas the nonoperative management of rotator cuff tears has been reported to have a success rate from 50 % to greater than 90 % [27–33], only a few studies have dealt with the outcome of nonoperative management of massive tears, specifically [28, 32]. Despite the general weakness and dysfunction of patients with massive rotator cuff tears, not every patient with a massive tear requires surgery. Moderately symptomatic patients may accept their functional limitations or have comorbidities that make them a less than ideal surgical candidate, and some tears are considered irreparable at the time of presentation [1].

By definition, an irreparable tear is one in which the defect cannot be closed intraoperatively or where closure of the tear during surgery is so challenging that it will almost certainly be associated with structural failure of the repair [19]. A number of studies have also suggested that if there are substantial lag signs present on clinical examination, if fatty infiltration of the respective muscles is beyond Goutallier stage 2 [12] and/or if there is superior migration of the humeral head resulting in an acromiohumeral distance of less than 7 mm [15], the probability of successful rotator cuff repair is so low that these tears can be deemed irreparable [19].

The purpose of this chapter is to outline the natural history of massive rotator cuff tears and to describe the role of nonoperative management.

Natural History

The natural history of massive rotator cuff tears is not well known [1]. However, there are a number of sequelae that develop as a result of massive tears. These sequelae are outlined below.

Tear Progression

In contrast to small rotator cuff tears with little or no retraction that frequently remain small [34], large and massive reparable tears usually increase

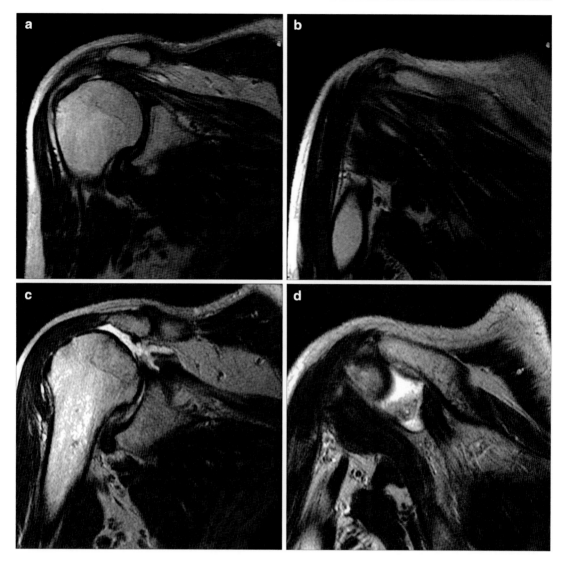

Fig. 4.1 Rotator cuff tear progression on sequential MRI studies. (**a**, **b**) Select coronal T2-weighted images demonstrate a medium-sized supraspinatus tear retracted to the mid-humeral head and without extension into the infraspinatus. (**c**, **d**) Select coronal T2-weighted images on fol- low-up MRI study performed approximately 1 year later demonstrate progression to a massive, irreparable tear involving both the supraspinatus and infraspinatus ten- dons with retraction to the glenoid rim

in size and can rapidly become irreparable with no further increase in pain or disability [1, 35].

A study by Zingg et al. [1] demonstrated that after a 4-year period of follow-up of massive rota- tor cuff tears, the size of the tendon tear increased, and fatty infiltration increased by approximately one stage in all three muscles. Moreover, four of the eight rotator cuff tears that were graded as

reparable at the time of diagnosis became irrepa- rable at the time of final follow-up (Fig. 4.1).

Therefore, it is critical to determine the defini- tive treatment of a massive, reparable tear at the time of its identification, taking into consider- ation the patient's symptoms, reparability of the lesion, and short- and longer-term functional demands [19].

Shoulder and Periscapular Kinematics

Massive tears can cause an uncoupling of forces across the glenohumeral joint and result in unstable shoulder kinematics, leading to a change in muscle activation patterns and coordination [36]. If shoulder kinematics can be maintained by the activation of other muscle groups, it is possible for the deltoid to compensate and allow continued functional overhead use of the arm [21]. This mechanism may explain asymptomatic massive rotator cuff tears [34, 37]. The preservation of teres minor is important for this compensation to occur, as teres minor is required for glenohumeral stability [38].

Due to the loss of the contribution of the supraspinatus in massive rotator cuff tears, the loss of abduction torque can only be compensated for by the use of the deltoid muscle. Relative to the supraspinatus, the deltoid can potentially generate a greater abduction torque, but the muscle force vector is more superiorly directed. With the lack of depressing and centralizing forces of the torn rotator cuff tendons, the consequence of this new deltoid muscle force vector is the superior shift of the reaction force and a dynamic upward glenohumeral subluxation [36, 38]. As a result, it becomes necessary for muscles with large adductor components, such as the pectoralis major and latissimus dorsi, to contract in order to provide glenohumeral stability. This "expensive" cocontraction is the only solution to generate net abduction torque [38]. However, it is likely that this cocontraction is also a cause for pain and the limitation in maximal arm elevation in patients with massive tears [39–41]. Steenbrink et al. [36] studied shoulder muscle activation in patients with massive rotator cuff tears, including the effects of subacromial pain suppression. They found that patients with massive rotator cuff tears were capable of arm abduction, but were actively hampered to do so due to pain [36, 41]. They also found that several depressor and adductor muscles (latissimus dorsi, pectoralis major, and teres major) shifted from generating adduction torque towards generating humeral head depression forces [36]. This increase in adductor muscle contraction was diminished to some extent after subacromial pain suppression.

Other studies have also demonstrated that massive cuff tears result in kinematic changes to multiple muscles that control scapulothoracic and scapulohumeral positions. Hawkes et al. [42] showed that in patients with massive cuff tears, EMG signal amplitudes were significantly higher in the biceps brachii, brachioradialis, upper trapezius, serratus anterior, latissimus dorsi, and teres major muscles.

Over time, patients may begin to fail to fully compensate for the destabilizing forces, and the overwhelming superiorly directed reaction force results in a static upward glenohumeral subluxation, also known as proximal migration of the humeral head [36]. This proximal migration of the humeral head is a common finding in symptomatic massive rotator cuff tears and represents a part of the natural history of tear progression [38].

Articular Cartilage

The abnormal joint mechanics secondary to massive cuff tears along with the superior migration of the humeral head result in significant alterations in articular surface contact pressures on both the glenoid and the humeral head [43]. These changes primarily affect the anterosuperior and anteroinferior glenoid, as well as the anteroinferior and the posterosuperior humeral head [43]. Reuther et al. [23] studied the effect of massive rotator cuff tears on glenohumeral articular cartilage in a rat model with a unilateral massive cuff tear. They found that massive tears led to decreased glenoid cartilage thickness in the anteroinferior region of the affected shoulders. In addition, equilibrium elastic modulus significantly decreased in the center, anterosuperior, anteroinferior, and superior regions. These results suggest that altered loading after rotator cuff injury may lead to damage to the joint with significant pain and dysfunction.

It is also postulated that articular cartilage nutrition is impaired both by synovial fluid leakage and by joint immobility, with resulting articular cartilage atrophy and subchondral osteoporosis.

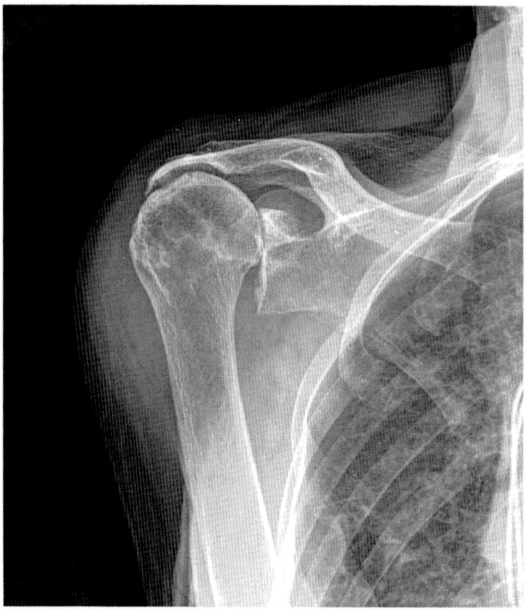

Fig. 4.2 Anteroposterior (AP) plain radiograph showing characteristic findings of rotator cuff tear arthropathy, with developing acetabularization of the acromion and femoralization of the humeral head secondary to superior migration of the humeral head

These factors combined contribute to the development of rotator cuff tear arthropathy, a term coined by Neer in 1977, who described the entity as a distinct form of glenohumeral arthritis associated with massive tears of the rotator cuff [25]. The end result of cuff tear arthropathy is the phenomenon of acetabularization of the acromion and femoralization of the humeral head, in which the articulation of the humeral head with the acromion from superior migration of the humeral head results in degenerative wear that creates cupping of the undersurface of the acromion (acetabularization) and rounding off of the humeral head (femoralization) (Fig. 4.2).

The Long Head of the Biceps Tendon (LHB)

The LHB also undergoes changes in massive rotator cuff tears. The LHB is believed to be a depressor or a dynamic stabilizer of the humeral head. Itoi et al. demonstrated that the biceps tendon

contributes not only to the superior-inferior stability of the humeral head but also to the anterior-posterior stability [44]. This role becomes more important in the presence of a rotator cuff tear [19, 45]. However, other studies have suggested that this stabilizing force is too small alone to stabilize the humeral head [46].

Sakurai et al. [47] studied the morphological changes of the LHB tendon in rotator cuff dysfunction in 170 cadavers. They found that in specimens with rotator cuff tears with a diameter less than 5 cm, stenosis at the bicipital groove induced by enlargement of the LHB occurred. In contrast, specimens with massive cuff tears (the longest diameter more than 5 cm) showed degenerative changes in the LHB as well as deficiency and wear in the medial wall of the groove, a potential cause of LHB instability. They suggested that the volume of the LHB increases in small tears to compensate for insufficient cuff function, which leads to stenosis of the bicipital groove, subsequently resulting in bicipital tendinitis. However, in massive cuff tears, the volume of the LHB decreases due to progressive wear of the LHB caused by the degenerative changes. Moreover, in specimens with massive cuff tears, medial instability of the LHB was common as a result of the decrease in height of the medial wall of the bicipital groove due to the extent of wear involving the subscapularis, including the soft tissues attached to the lesser tubercle. Therefore, LHB changes and degeneration are considered an important cause of shoulder pain in the setting of massive rotator cuff tears. Although it is often difficult to differentiate pain due to LHB changes from rotator cuff tear pain, it is an important consideration as LHB tenotomy or tenodesis may provide substantial relief and improvement [19, 21, 48, 49].

The Deltoid

Massive rotator cuff tears have been implicated as a cause of deltoid tears. Although tears of the deltoid muscle in patients without prior surgical intervention are quite rare, there have been reports that massive rotator cuff tears can lead to attritional deltoid muscle or tendon tears over

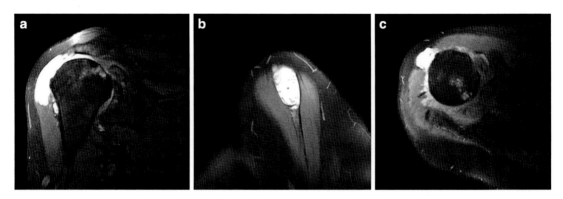

Fig. 4.3 Select (**a**) coronal, (**b**) sagittal, and (**c**) axial T2-weighted MRI images demonstrate rupture of the middle deltoid in a patient with a massive, irreparable rotator cuff tear. It has been speculated that proximal migration of the humeral head associated with massive, irreparable rotator cuff tears results in attritional tearing of the deltoid from friction between the greater tuberosity and the deltoid origin on the acromion

time [50, 51] (Fig. 4.3). The exact etiology of these deltoid tears is not clearly known. Yet, it has been speculated that the proximal migration of the humeral head associated with massive cuff tears results in friction between the greater tuberosity and the undersurface of the myotendinous junction of the deltoid, with resultant stretching and fraying of the deltoid muscle fibers that progressively weakens the muscle and eventually causes rupture [50]. This theory is supported by the fact that reported deltoid partial thickness tears involve the undersurface of the deltoid [51]. These partial thickness tears leak bursal fluid into the deltoid muscle belly resulting in intramuscular cyst formation described by Ilaslan et al. [51].

Blazar et al. [50] reported on a series of patients with spontaneous detachment of the acromial origin of the deltoid. All patients had chronic massive rotator cuff tears and were older than 65 years of age (mean 73 years). The majority of the patients were women. All patients described a sudden onset of weakness consistent with an acute deltoid detachment, and physical examination showed involvement of the middle deltoid and a characteristic defect at the acromion, a defect that became pronounced with attempted elevation of the arm. Using MRI, Ilaslan et al. [51] also demonstrated that the anterior deltoid can be involved and stressed the importance of the coracoacromial arch in providing superior restraint to the humeral head in the setting of a massive rotator cuff tear.

Erosion or stress fracture of the acromion has also been reported in chronic massive cuff tears as a result of the superior migration of the humeral head and progressive wear along the undersurface of the acromion [52] (Fig. 4.4). The dynamic anterosuperior dislocation of the humeral head, known as anterior-superior escape, has also been implicated as a cause of erosion and fracture of the acromion and attritional changes to the anterior deltoid [51].

Nonoperative Treatment of Massive Rotator Cuff Tears

The management of massive rotator cuff tears is complex due to the many involved variables. The goal of the treatment is focused on pain reduction and functional improvements [23]. Unfortunately, the published literature does not contain enough data to allow establishment of an evidence-based, universally acceptable treatment algorithm for massive rotator cuff tears [19]. Furthermore, the value of nonoperative treatment is not well established, and there is no evidence that nonoperative treatment substantially alters the course or natural history of massive tears [17, 28, 31, 53–55].

Nonoperative management of massive rotator cuff tears is typically reserved for patients whose symptoms do not involve debilitating pain or in whom surgical intervention is contraindicated. It involves a combination of activity modification,

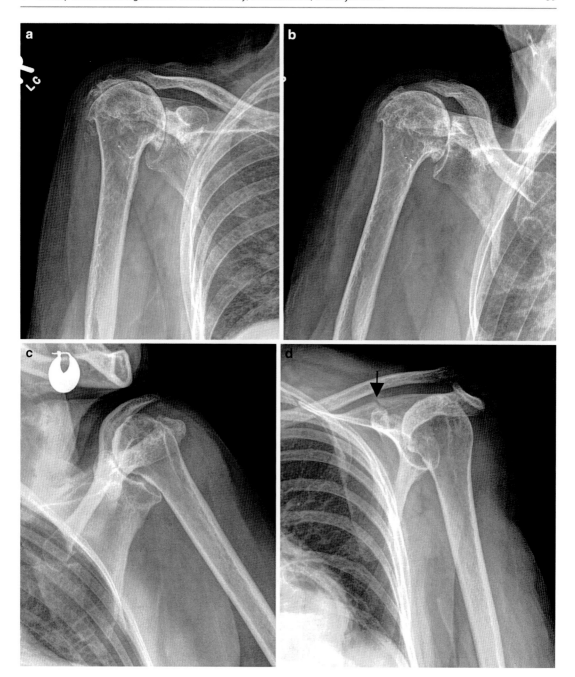

Fig. 4.4 Examples of acromial erosion and stress fractures in patients with massive, irreparable rotator cuff tears. (**a**, **b**) Anteroposterior (AP) plain radiographs of an advanced case of rotator cuff tear arthropathy demonstrate acetabularization of the acromion and femoralization of the humeral head, as well as the development of acromial fragmentation and erosion from progressive bony wear. (**c**, **d**) Anteroposterior (AP) plain radiographs show the development of a stress fracture along the scapular spine at the base of the acromion (**d**, *arrow*) in a patient with significant superior wear of the glenoid and medialization of the humeral head from rotator cuff tear arthropathy

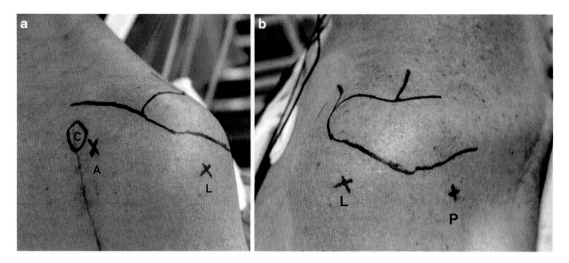

Fig. 4.5 Skin locations of anterior, posterior, and lateral cortisone injections. (**a**) An anterior injection (marked *A*) is performed in the location of a standard anterior arthroscopic portal, at a point just lateral to the tip of the coracoid process (marked *C*), in the natural soft spot created by the glenohumeral joint. (**a**, **b**) A lateral injection (marked *L*) is performed in the location of a standard lat- eral arthroscopic portal, approximately 2–3 cm distal to the lateral edge of the acromion, along the anterior aspect of the bone. (**b**) A posterior injection (marked *P*) is typi- cally performed in the location of a standard posterior arthroscopic portal, at a point approximately 1–2 cm medial and 2–3 cm distal to the posterolateral corner of the acromion

nonsteroidal anti-inflammatories (NSAIDs), steroid injections, physical therapy with emphasis on training the anterior deltoid muscle, and other alternative treatment methods. Other goals of therapy include reeducation of muscle recruitment, coordination of muscle cocontraction, periscapu- lar strengthening, maintenance of motion, and improvement of proprioception [21]. Therapy should be altered based on the specific patient complaints, as some patients may have pain pri- marily from loss of function and strength due to their massive rotator cuff tear, while others may have pain related to stiffness that has developed from arthritic changes or the occurrence of an adhesive capsulitis.

NSAIDs help with both pain control and reduction of inflammation and thus are thought to improve function. These medications can be taken as needed in over-the-counter or prescrip- tion doses. More extended use of NSAIDs should be closely monitored for potential side effects, including gastrointestinal discomfort or bleeding, and renal or cardiac abnormalities. Oral narcotics may also be used to reduce more severe, acute pain from massive rotator cuff tears, such as after an acute injury. However, we do not recommend

the use of narcotics for pain control, as they can be associated with nausea, vomiting, and constipation, and more extended use can lead to problems with drug tolerance and dependence.

Steroid injections are also thought to be an effective nonoperative treatment modality in patients with massive rotator cuff tears because of their strong anti-inflammatory effect, with the ability to locally decrease inflammation in the shoulder caused by the rotator cuff tear and/or associated degenerative changes, resulting in decreased pain and improvement in function. This effect can be stronger and more long lasting than the anti-inflammatory response of an oral NSAID. Due to the massive size of the rotator cuff tear, a subacromial steroid injection also becomes an intra-articular injection in these patients. Therefore, the injection can be performed from any approach, including anterior, posterior, or lat- eral (Fig. 4.5). The desired approach should be determined based on clinician preference, bony anatomy, and patient body habitus.

A posterior injection is typically performed in the location of a standard posterior arthroscopic por- tal (Fig. 4.5). This point is approximately 1–2 cm medial and 2–3 cm distal to the posterolateral corner of the acromion; however, the location can vary based on patient body habitus. Aiming the needle just under the acromion will direct the injection subacromially, while pointing the needle deeper and in the direction of the coracoid process anteriorly will guide the injection more directly into the glenohumeral joint. An anterior injection may provide easier access to the glenohumeral joint in a larger patient, as the soft tissue distance the needle must traverse is less because of the deltopectoral interval and rotator interval. This injection is performed in the location of a standard anterior arthroscopic portal, at a point just lateral to the tip of the coracoid process, in the natural soft spot created by the glenohumeral joint (Fig. 4.5). Finally, a lateral injection provides access to the subacromial space. This injection is performed in the location of a standard lateral arthroscopic portal, approximately 2–3 cm distal to the lateral edge of the acromion, along the anterior aspect of the bone (Fig. 4.5). In a patient with superior migration of the humeral head and a decreased acromiohumeral interval, this point may be a more difficult approach for injection, and an anterior or posterior approach may be preferred. Regardless of the chosen injection location, confirmation of correct needle position is made by the ease with which the steroid is injected. If substantial resistance is felt while trying to perform an injection, the needle should be repositioned until fluid from the syringe can be easily injected without resistance.

The primary benefit of steroid injections is pain relief, which may also improve shoulder function due to the loss of pain inhibition and increase the ability to participate in therapy. Side effects can rarely occur, including an allergic reaction to one of the injection ingredients, skin depigmentation at the injection site, infection, bleeding, and elevation of blood sugar levels in diabetic patients (see Pearls and Pitfalls of Steroid Injections). Muscle or tendon rupture is also possible if the steroid is inadvertently injected while in an intramuscular or intratendinous position.

Viscosupplementation injections with hyaluronate, as well as platelet-rich plasma (PRP) injections, have also been described in the nonoperative treatment of rotator cuff tears, but with minimal supporting evidence to date. Finally, alternative treatment methods such as electric, shock wave, laser, and acupuncture therapies have been described.

Indications

Since there is no evidence that the results of biceps tenotomy or tenodesis, subacromial decompression with debridement, partial rotator cuff repair, tendon transfer, or reverse total shoulder arthroplasty are strongly dependent on the timing between tendon rupture and treatment, it is reasonable that irreparable rotator cuff tears be initially treated with nonoperative management [19]. Therefore, all patients with a massive irreparable rotator cuff tear are candidates for nonoperative treatment. Any of the nonoperative treatment modalities may be pursued, either sequentially or in combination. Often a combined approach of activity modification, use of NSAIDs and/or steroid injections, and physical therapy may provide more substantial symptomatic benefit than any one treatment alone. The decision to pursue one or more treatment modalities is based on the severity of the patient's symptoms and dysfunction.

Contraindications

There are no true contraindications to nonoperative treatment of massive rotator cuff tears. However, in a study by Zingg et al. [1], a substantial structural deterioration of the glenohumeral joint and the rotator cuff tendons was radiographically found over a period of 4 years, despite the good clinical results of nonoperative treatment. Glenohumeral osteoarthritis progressed by one to two grades, meaning that joint-preserving surgical procedures such as a latissimus dorsi transfer for a posterosuperior rotator cuff tear or a pectoralis major transfer for an anterosuperior rotator cuff tear, would have been less likely to succeed. There was also a significant decrease in the acromiohumeral distance and MRI-defined fatty muscle infiltration progressed by approximately one stage in each of the three rotator cuff muscles [1, 56]. The progression of rotator cuff pathology represented by these two findings is concerning for a reparable massive rotator cuff tear becoming irreparable over time with nonoperative management [1]. Therefore, it is crucial to disclose this possibility of tear progression to patients with a reparable massive rotator cuff tear upon presentation. Initial nonoperative treatment may not be indicated for massive reparable tears in patients with high midterm to long-term functional demands, unless the patient has significant medical comorbidities that would outweigh the benefits of surgery [19].

Contraindications may exist for specific treatment modalities. Patients with stomach ulcers, bleeding disorders, diabetes, renal compromise, significant cardiac history, multiple medical comorbidities, hypertension, and those on anticoagulation should discuss the use of NSAIDs with their primary care physician prior to starting one of these medications, as NSAIDs may be associated with significant side effects in these patients.

With regard to steroid or other local injections, patients with an allergy to any of the ingredients of the injections should not receive them. In addition, steroid injections should not be performed in or around a shoulder if there is any concern for infection. Those patients on anticoagulation may not be able to safely undergo an injection because of the potential bleeding risk. Finally, steroid injections can raise blood sugar levels in diabetic patients. It is important to discuss this possibility with these patients and have them closely monitor blood sugar levels after an injection. In a poorly controlled diabetic, it may be a reason to avoid an injection.

If a steroid injection provides substantial benefit, most clinicians recommend waiting a minimum of 3–4 months before repeating an injection and even longer if symptoms are not severe enough to warrant it. Some authors have suggested that repeated steroid injections can play a role in the development of deltoid ruptures, as intratendinous injections have been shown to have adverse effects [51]. There is also concern that repeated injections may eventually weaken the remaining rotator cuff tissue.

Outcomes of Nonoperative Treatment of Massive Rotator Cuff Tears

Only a small number of studies have investigated the outcomes of nonoperative treatment for massive rotator cuff tears. It is important to note that some of these studies may have a patient selection bias, as patients with high functional demands or unacceptable pain complaints are more likely to undergo surgery and can be excluded from a nonoperative analysis. Therefore, the conclusions of some of these studies may only apply to elderly patients with lower functional demands and may not be generalizable to all patients with a massive rotator cuff tear, especially those with higher functional demands.

A number of studies have reported on the outcomes of nonoperative management of full-thickness rotator cuff tears as a whole, with variable results and successful outcomes ranging from 50 to 90 % [27–33]. Although these reports are not specific to massive rotator cuff tears, they may still provide some insight into outcomes with these tears. These studies show a large variability in the specific nonoperative treatments that are utilized, including the type and amount of physical therapy given, the use and frequency of NSAIDs and/or steroid injections, and the types of additional modalities used, if any. Some studies have suggested that full-thickness rotator cuff tears treated with nonoperative modalities provide inferior outcomes for patients whose symptoms have been chronic in nature [21]. For example, Bokor et al. [28] studied nonoperative treatment using NSAIDs, stretching, strengthening, and occasional steroid injections in 53 patients with full-thickness rotator cuff tears at an average 7.6-year follow-up. They found that a satisfactory outcome occurred in 24 of 28 patients (86 %) who presented early, whereas only 9 of 16 patients (56 %) seen after 6 months of symptoms achieved a satisfactory outcome. They also demonstrated that functional capacity and range of motion did not improve to the same extent as the resolution of pain [28]. Itoi et al. [32] reported on the nonoperative management of 124 shoulders in 114 patients with full-thickness rotator cuff tears at an average follow-up of 3.4 years.

Treatment included a combination of rest, NSAIDs, local anesthetic and/or steroid injections, active and passive range of motion, and muscle strengthening. They determined that patients with more than 1 year of persistent symptoms showed no significant increase in functional scores at final follow-up, and patients observed more than 6 years showed significantly lower scores than those with a shorter follow-up period. Therefore, nonoperative treatment may be most effective when applied in the early phase of symptoms, with satisfactory short- and midterm results, but potentially less satisfactory results at longer-term follow-up. Moreover, the authors showed that patients with preserved range of motion and strength at the time of initiation of treatment, regardless of severity of pain, had better functional scores than their counterparts [32].

With regard to studies specific to the outcomes of nonoperative treatment of massive rotator cuff tears, Ainsworth reported on ten patients with massive rotator cuff tears, defined on ultrasound as a tear in which the leading edge had retracted past the glenoid margin, who were treated with a physical therapy program. The program was designed to help with patient education, posture correction, muscle recruitment, stretching, strengthening, proprioception, and adaptation. The author observed significantly improved function over a 12-week period in the Oxford Shoulder Disability and Short Form 36-Item Health Survey scores [57].

A recent study by Zingg et al. [1] in 19 patients with massive rotator cuff tears documented surprisingly good clinical outcomes at mean 4-year follow-up using nonoperative treatment, but with substantial structural deterioration of cartilage, tendon, and muscle over time, as noted above. Nonoperative treatment included a standardized rehabilitation program and/or pain medication (systemic and local NSAIDs, as well as subacromial steroid injections) or no treatment. These patients demonstrated mild pain with no appreciable change in their active motion and were able to maintain satisfactory shoulder function over time. The mean relative constant score was 83 %, and the mean subjective shoulder value was 68 %. The score for pain averaged 11.5 points on a 0 to 15-point visual analogue scale in which 15 points represented no pain. Active range of motion did not deteriorate over time, with a significant increase of 24° in forward flexion. At final follow-up, forward flexion and abduction averaged 136°; external rotation, 39°; and internal rotation, 66°. Of the six patients who presented with pseudoparalysis of the shoulder (defined in the study as active flexion of <90° with full passive motion), five had a traumatic rotator cuff tear and regained good range of motion after nonoperative therapy, whereas the one patient with a chronic rotator cuff tear continued to demonstrate pseudoparalysis at the time of final follow-up.

Despite the good clinical outcomes in this study, all patients showed a progression of glenohumeral osteoarthritis, a decrease in the acromiohumeral distance, an increase in the size of the rotator cuff tear, and an increase in fatty infiltration by a mean of one stage in all three muscles. Four of the eight rotator cuff tears that were considered reparable at the time of presentation became irreparable at the time of final follow-up. Moreover, patients with a three-tendon tear showed more progression of osteoarthritis than did patients with a two-tendon tear [1]. Although the patients in this series had less abduction strength compared with the strength reported after successful repairs of massive rotator cuff tears [8], the average strength of 3 kg did not seem to restrict the daily activities of moderately symptomatic patients with relatively low functional demands. The authors concluded that patients with nonoperatively managed, moderately symptomatic massive rotator cuff tears can maintain satisfactory shoulder function for at least 4 years despite significant progression of degenerative structural joint changes.

There are no studies that report on the effectiveness of NSAIDs alone as a nonoperative treatment in massive rotator cuff tears. NSAIDs have been found to be more effective than placebo in improving function and decreasing pain in patients with rotator cuff tendinosis, but no studies have been reported in rotator cuff tears.

With regard to the effectiveness of steroid injections in massive rotator cuff tears, there are mixed reports on the outcomes, especially with regard to pain control. Many studies have found a benefit, yet two studies reported no additional benefit [27, 58]. Vad et al. [59] studied the effects of nonoperative treatment for massive rotator cuff tears with or without steroid injection, at an average follow-up of 3.2 years. They found that the steroid injection group had significantly better pain and total scores and significantly shorter time to regain maximal range of motion when compared with the group that did not receive a steroid injection. The combination of steroid injections and physical therapy was superior to physical therapy alone, with an excellent or good outcome in 65 % of patients in the no injection group and 75 % in the injection group [59]. Both groups reached the same maximal range of motion, but patients receiving a combination of steroid injection and physical therapy achieved maximal range of motion at an average of 5.3 months after treatment was begun versus 9.3 months in patients receiving physical therapy alone [59].

One randomized trial [60] involving patients with full-thickness rotator cuff tears examined the effects of intra-articular steroid injection versus hyaluronate injection in patients also undergoing nonoperative treatment with NSAIDs and physical therapy. No difference was seen with respect to satisfaction of treatment between the two groups at 24-week follow-up. Despite enthusiasm regarding the use of PRP injections in nonoperative rotator cuff tear treatment, there is little data to recommend for or against its use. One double-blinded randomized control trial comparing subacromial PRP injections to placebo saline subacromial injections has recently been reported for the nonoperative treatment of chronic rotator cuff tendinopathy [61]. All patients underwent a 6-week therapy program in combination with the injections. At 1-year follow-up, both groups showed significant functional improvement, but the PRP injections were no more effective in improving quality of life, pain, disability, and shoulder range of motion than the placebo saline injections. Further high-quality evidence is needed to better define the use of PRP injections in management of rotator cuff pathology.

There are no studies on the use of alternative treatment methods such as electric, shock wave, laser, or acupuncture therapy in the management of massive rotator cuff tears. These treatment methods have been studied in rotator cuff tendinosis, but not in rotator cuff tears.

Prognostic Factors for Treatment

Vad et al. [59] analyzed the results of management of 108 patients with massive rotator cuff tears treated both operatively and nonoperatively. The authors demonstrated that poor outcomes in the nonsurgical treatment group were associated with the presence of three or more of the following negative prognostic factors:

1. External rotation and abduction strength less than grade 3/5 on the MRC scale
2. Presence of muscle atrophy
3. Decreased passive range of motion
4. Presence of glenohumeral osteoarthritis
5. Superior migration of the humeral head

Patients in the surgical treatment groups in this study (arthroscopic debridement or rotator cuff repair) with these negative prognostic factors also had poor outcomes.

Conclusions

The natural history of massive rotator cuff tears is not well known. Nonoperative treatment is successful in decreasing pain in a large number of patients in short- to midterm follow-up, especially lower-demand patients. Patient function with nonoperative treatment is highly dependent on their pretreatment range of motion and function. Physical therapy should focus on strengthening of the anterior deltoid and any remaining anterior and posterior rotator cuff muscles. The addition of steroid injections to the nonoperative treatment approach does seem to offer additional benefit in regard to pain reduction. Nonoperative treatment, however, does not prevent the development of degenerative changes in the glenohumeral joint and tear progression, including an increase in fatty infiltration and muscle atrophy. Therefore, outcomes may deteriorate over time.

References

1. Zingg PO, Jost B, Sukthankar A, Buhler M, Pfirrmann CW, Gerber C. Clinical and structural outcomes of nonoperative management of massive rotator cuff tears. J Bone Joint Surg Am. 2007;89(9):1928–34.

2. Uhthoff HK, Sarkar K. An algorithm for shoulder pain caused by soft-tissue disorders. Clin Orthop Relat Res. 1990;254:121–7.

3. Yamamoto A, Takagishi K, Osawa T, Yanagawa T, Nakajima D, Shitara H, et al. Prevalence and risk factors of a rotator cuff tear in the general population. J Shoulder Elbow Surg. 2010;19(1):116–20.

4. Codman EA. Rupture of the supraspinatus tendon. 1911. Clin Orthop Relat Res. 1990;254:3–26.

5. Wening JD, Hollis RF, Hughes RE, Kuhn JE. Quantitative morphology of full thickness rotator cuff tears. Clin Anat. 2002;15(1):18–22.

6. Steinbacher P, Tauber M, Kogler S, Stoiber W, Resch H, Sanger AM. Effects of rotator cuff ruptures on the cellular and intracellular composition of the human supraspinatus muscle. Tissue Cell. 2010;42(1):37–41.

7. Bigliani LU, Cordasco FA, McLlveen SJ, Musso ES. Operative repair of massive rotator cuff tears: Long-term results. J Shoulder Elbow Surg. 1992;1(3):120–30.

8. Gerber C, Fuchs B, Hodler J. The results of repair of massive tears of the rotator cuff. J Bone Joint Surg Am. 2000;82(4):505–15.

9. Zumstein MA, Jost B, Hempel J, Hodler J, Gerber C. The clinical and structural long-term results of open repair of massive tears of the rotator cuff. J Bone Joint Surg Am. 2008;90(11):2423–31.

10. Meyer DC, Lajtai G, von Rechenberg B, Pfirrmann CW, Gerber C. Tendon retracts more than muscle in experimental chronic tears of the rotator cuff. J Bone Joint Surg Br. 2006;88(11):1533–8.

11. Hersche O, Gerber C. Passive tension in the supraspinatus musculotendinous unit after long-standing rupture of its tendon: a preliminary report. J Shoulder Elbow Surg. 1998;7(4):393–6.

12. Goutallier D, Postel JM, Bernageau J, Lavau L, Voisin MC. Fatty muscle degeneration in cuff ruptures. Pre- and postoperative evaluation by CT scan. Clin Orthop Relat Res. 1994;304:78–83.

13. Gruber G, Bernhardt GA, Clar H, Zacherl M, Glehr M, Wurnig C. Measurement of the acromiohumeral interval on standardized anteroposterior radiographs: a prospective study of observer variability. J Shoulder Elbow Surg. 2010;19(1):10–3.

14. Hamada K, Fukuda H, Mikasa M, Kobayashi Y. Roentgenographic findings in massive rotator cuff tears. A long-term observation. Clin Orthop Relat Res. 1990;254:92–6.

15. Walch G, Marechal E, Maupas J, Liotard JP. Surgical treatment of rotator cuff rupture. Prognostic factors. Rev Chir Orthop Reparatrice Appar Mot. 1992;78(6):379–88.

16. Weiner DS, Macnab I. Superior migration of the humeral head. A radiological aid in the diagnosis of tears of the rotator cuff. J Bone Joint Surg Br. 1970;52(3):524–7.

17. Milgrom C, Schaffler M, Gilbert S, van Holsbeeck M. Rotator-cuff changes in asymptomatic adults. The effect of age, hand dominance and gender. J Bone Joint Surg Br. 1995;77(2):296–8.

18. Sher JS, Uribe JW, Posada A, Murphy BJ, Zlatkin MB. Abnormal findings on magnetic resonance images of asymptomatic shoulders. J Bone Joint Surg Am. 1995;77(1):10–5.

19. Gerber C, Wirth SH, Farshad M. Treatment options for massive rotator cuff tears. J Shoulder Elbow Surg. 2011;20(2 Suppl):S20–9.

20. Itoi E, Minagawa H, Sato T, Sato K, Tabata S. Isokinetic strength after tears of the supraspinatus tendon. J Bone Joint Surg Br. 1997;79(1):77–82.

21. Neri BR, Chan KW, Kwon YW. Management of massive and irreparable rotator cuff tears. J Shoulder Elbow Surg. 2009;18(5):808–18.

22. Burkhart SS. Arthroscopic treatment of massive rotator cuff tears. Clin Orthop Relat Res. 2001;390:107–18.

23. Reuther KE, Sarver JJ, Schultz SM, Lee CS, Sehgal CM, Glaser DL, et al. Glenoid cartilage mechanical properties decrease after rotator cuff tears in a rat model. J Orthop Res. 2012;30(9):1435–9.

24. Hsu HC, Luo ZP, Stone JJ, Huang TH, An KN. Correlation between rotator cuff tear and glenohumeral degeneration. Acta Orthop Scand. 2003;74(1):89–94.

25. Neer 2nd CS, Craig EV, Fukuda H. Cuff-tear arthropathy. J Bone Joint Surg Am. 1983;65(9):1232–44.

26. Petersson CJ. Degeneration of the gleno-humeral joint. An anatomical study. Acta orthopaedica Scandinavica. 1983;54(2):277–83.

27. Bartolozzi A, Andreychik D, Ahmad S. Determinants of outcome in the treatment of rotator cuff disease. Clin Orthop Relat Res. 1994;308:90–7.

28. Bokor DJ, Hawkins RJ, Huckell GH, Angelo RL, Schickendantz MS. Results of nonoperative management of full-thickness tears of the rotator cuff. Clin Orthop Relat Res. 1993;294:103–10.

29. Brown JT. Early assessment of supraspinatus tears; procaine infiltration as a guide to treatment. J Bone Joint Surg. 1949;31B(3):423–5.

30. Cofield RH. Rotator cuff disease of the shoulder. J Bone Joint Surg Am. 1985;67(6):974–9.

31. Hawkins RH, Dunlop R. Nonoperative treatment of rotator cuff tears. Clin Orthop Relat Res. 1995;321:178–88.

32. Itoi E, Tabata S. Conservative treatment of rotator cuff tears. Clin Orthop Relat Res. 1992;275:165–73.

33. Samilson RL, Binder WF. Symptomatic full thickness tears of rotator cuff. An analysis of 292 shoulders in 276 patients. Orthop Clin North Am. 1975;6(2):449–66.

34. Yamaguchi K, Tetro AM, Blam O, Evanoff BA, Teefey SA, Middleton WD. Natural history of asymptomatic rotator cuff tears: a longitudinal analysis of asymptomatic tears detected sonographically. J Shoulder Elbow Surg. 2001;10(3):199–203.

35. Zvijac JE, Levy HJ, Lemak LJ. Arthroscopic subacromial decompression in the treatment of full thickness rotator cuff tears: a 3- to 6-year follow-up. Arthroscopy. 1994;10(5):518–23.
36. Steenbrink F, de Groot JH, Veeger HE, Meskers CG, van de Sande MA, Rozing PM. Pathological muscle activation patterns in patients with massive rotator cuff tears, with and without subacromial anaesthetics. Man Ther. 2006;11(3):231–7.
37. Kelly BT, Williams RJ, Cordasco FA, Backus SI, Otis JC, Weiland DE, et al. Differential patterns of muscle activation in patients with symptomatic and asymptomatic rotator cuff tears. J Shoulder Elbow Surg. 2005;14(2):165–71.
38. Steenbrink F, de Groot JH, Veeger HE, van der Helm FC, Rozing PM. Glenohumeral stability in simulated rotator cuff tears. J Biomech. 2009;42(11):1740–5.
39. Iannotti JP, Hennigan S, Herzog R, Kella S, Kelley M, Leggin B, et al. Latissimus dorsi tendon transfer for irreparable posterosuperior rotator cuff tears. Factors affecting outcome. J Bone Joint Surg Am. 2006;88(2):342–8.
40. Jost B, Pfirrmann CW, Gerber C, Switzerland Z. Clinical outcome after structural failure of rotator cuff repairs. J Bone Joint Surg Am. 2000;82(3):304–14.
41. de Groot JH, van de Sande MA, Meskers CG, Rozing PM. Pathological Teres Major activation in patients with massive rotator cuff tears alters with pain relief and/or salvage surgery transfer. Clinical Biomech. 2006;21 Suppl 1:S27–32.
42. Hawkes DH, Alizadehkhaiyat O, Kemp GJ, Fisher AC, Roebuck MM, Frostick SP. Shoulder muscle activation and coordination in patients with a massive rotator cuff tear: an electromyographic study. J Orthop Res. 2012;30(7):1140–6.
43. Feeney MS, O'Dowd J, Kay EW, Colville J. Glenohumeral articular cartilage changes in rotator cuff disease. J Shoulder Elbow Surg. 2003;12(1):20–3.
44. Itoi E, Motzkin NE, Morrey BF, An KN. Stabilizing function of the long head of the biceps in the hanging arm position. J Shoulder Elbow Surg. 1994;3(3):135–42.
45. Kumar VP, Satku K, Balasubramaniam P. The role of the long head of biceps brachii in the stabilization of the head of the humerus. Clin Orthop Relat Res. 1989;244:172–5.
46. Perry J, Bekey GA. EMG-force relationships in skeletal muscle. Crit Rev Biomed Eng. 1981;7(1):1–22.
47. Sakurai G, Ozaki J, Tomita Y, Nakagawa Y, Kondo T, Tamai S. Morphologic changes in long head of biceps brachii in rotator cuff dysfunction. J Orthop Sci. 1998;3(3):137–42.
48. Boileau P, Baque F, Valerio L, Ahrens P, Chuinard C, Trojani C. Isolated arthroscopic biceps tenotomy or tenodesis improves symptoms in patients with massive irreparable rotator cuff tears. J Bone Joint Surg Am. 2007;89(4):747–57.
49. Walch G, Edwards TB, Boulahia A, Nove-Josserand L, Neyton L, Szabo I. Arthroscopic tenotomy of the long head of the biceps in the treatment of rotator cuff tears: clinical and radiographic results of 307 cases. J Shoulder Elbow Surg. 2005;14(3):238–46.
50. Blazar PE, Williams GR, Iannotti JP. Spontaneous detachment of the deltoid muscle origin. J Shoulder Elbow Surg. 1998;7(4):389–92.
51. Ilaslan H, Iannotti JP, Recht MP. Deltoid muscle and tendon tears in patients with chronic rotator cuff tears. Skeletal Radiol. 2007;36(6):503–7.
52. Morisawa K, Yamashita K, Asami A, Nishikawa H, Watanabe H. Spontaneous rupture of the deltoid muscle associated with massive tearing of the rotator cuff. J Shoulder Elbow Surg. 1997;6(6):556–8.
53. Ainsworth R, Lewis JS. Exercise therapy for the conservative management of full thickness tears of the rotator cuff: a systematic review. Br J Sports Med. 2007;41(4):200–10.
54. Goldberg BA, Nowinski RJ, Matsen 3rd FA. Outcome of nonoperative management of full-thickness rotator cuff tears. Clin Orthop Relat Res. 2001;382:99–107.
55. Wirth MA, Basamania C, Rockwood Jr CA. Nonoperative management of full-thickness tears of the rotator cuff. Orthop Clin North Am. 1997;28(1):59–67.
56. Meyer DC, Hoppeler H, von Rechenberg B, Gerber C. A pathomechanical concept explains muscle loss and fatty muscular changes following surgical tendon release. J Orthop Sci. 2004;22(5):1004–7.
57. Ainsworth R. Physiotherapy rehabilitation in patients with massive, irreparable rotator cuff tears. Musculoskeletal Care. 2006;4(3):140–51.
58. Darlington LG, Coomes EN. The effects of local steroid injection for supraspinatus tears. Rheumatol Rehabil. 1977;16(3):172–9.
59. Vad VB, Warren RF, Altchek DW, O'Brien SJ, Rose HA, Wickiewicz TL. Negative prognostic factors in managing massive rotator cuff tears. Clin J Sport Med. 2002;12(3):151–7.
60. Shibata Y, Midorikawa K, Emoto G, Naito M. Clinical evaluation of sodium hyaluronate for the treatment of patients with rotator cuff tear. J Shoulder Elbow Surg. 2001;10(3):209–16.
61. Kesikburun S, Tan AK, Yilmaz B, Yasar E, Yazicioglu K. Platelet-rich plasma injections in the treatment of chronic rotator cuff tendinopathy: a randomized controlled trial with 1-Year follow-up. Am J Sports Med. 2013;41:2609–16.

Arthroscopic Treatment

5

Anthony Ho and Andrew S. Neviaser

Pearls and Pitfalls

Pearls

- Any tear that should be repaired can be repaired arthroscopically.
- The goals of arthroscopic repair are the same as repairs done open, a tension-free reconstruction of the native footprint.
- Arthroscopic portals can be made in any position where there is no neurovascular structure. The surgeon should not feel constrained to using only named portals.
- Physician-directed therapy is critical to the outcome and should be dictated by tissue quality, tear size, and patient age.

Pitfalls

- Tears with significant muscular fatty infiltration or atrophy are unlikely to heal even if repair is possible.
- Over-tensioning a repair to achieve a double-row or transosseous equivalent repair will likely lead to failure.

- Subscapularis tears can be easily missed if the insertion is not carefully examined.
- In massive tears, early motion therapy should be avoided to protect the repair. Early stiffness may result but will resolve.

Introduction

The treatment of massive rotator cuff tears presents both technical and biological challenges for shoulder surgeons. Although the early arthroscopic treatment of massive tears resulted in high re-tear rates [1], advances in arthroscopic instrumentation and better patient selection have improved outcomes. Now, the critical question guiding treatment is not whether a tear can be repaired, but whether repair of a torn rotator cuff will lead to a predictable outcome. This question is best answered by assessing prognostic variables such as patient age, fatty infiltration or atrophy of the cuff musculature, and size of the tear, rather than whether the repair is done open or arthroscopically. Any tear that should be repaired can be repaired arthroscopically, and arthroscopy provides several advantages over the traditional open or mini-open techniques. In arthroscopy, the surgeon is not constrained by a single incision, allowing improved visualization of large tears. There is less surgical trauma to the deltoid,

A. Ho, MD (✉) • A.S. Neviaser, MD
Department of Orthopaedic Surgery,
George Washington University Hospital,
2150 Pennsylvania Avenue, NW, Room 7-416,
Washington, DC 20037, USA
e-mail: agh124@gwu.edu; aneviaser@gmail.com

L.V. Gulotta and E.V. Craig (eds.), *Massive Rotator Cuff Tears: Diagnosis and Management*,
DOI 10.1007/978-1-4899-7494-5_5, © Springer Science+Business Media New York 2015

and the potential complication of deltoid dehiscence seen after some open approaches is avoided. Like other types of complex surgery, experience is a critical factor when considering treatment of massive tears. Surgeons should be proficient in repairing small tears before the repair of large or massive tears is attempted via an arthroscopic approach.

Although the majority of patients with massive tears are best served with complete repair, older patients or those with high-grade fatty infiltration may have a more predictable outcome with limited treatments such as simple debridement of the rotator cuff and release of the long head of the biceps. The following chapter serves to describe the appropriate evaluation and treatment of massive rotator cuff tears using arthroscopic techniques.

Classification

There are several ways of defining massive rotator cuff tears. Both functional and anatomic characteristics have been used, but each has their own limitations. Cofield et al. [2] defined a massive tear as any tear pattern with a diameter greater than 5 cm. Burkhart [3] used a similar definition but included that a portion of the superior humeral head remained uncovered. Zumstein et al. [4] provided a more functional interpretation, describing massive tears as those extending completely through at least two rotator cuff tendons.

Tear location can also be useful in describing these defects. Most tears fall into one of two distinct anatomic patterns: anterosuperior and posterosuperior. Posterosuperior tears, which include the supraspinatus and infraspinatus, are more common [5]. Anterosuperior tears, which involve the supraspinatus and subscapularis tendons, are less common but are more commonly associated with anterosuperior escape of the humeral head if the coracoacromial arch is violated.

Burkhart and Lo [6] formulated a classification system based on tear pattern. Crescent-shaped tears are small tears that are commonly seen in routine rotator cuff repairs. They have medial-lateral mobility and can often be repaired directly to the tuberosity. U-shaped tears have a central portion of tendon that has retracted medially, often at or past the glenoid rim. Recognition of this subtype is important since repair of the tendon directly to the tuberosity results in high tensile stresses across the repair, potentially resulting in overload and failure. Margin convergence can be effective in these cases and will be described later. L-shaped tears have both transverse and longitudinal components, creating two separate leaflets that retract medially. Massive, contracted, immobile tears comprise the last group that may require extensive releases to restore sufficient mobility to the tendon.

Radiographic Evaluation

Imaging studies play a critical role in not only the diagnosis of massive rotator cuff tears but also in the selection of appropriate treatment. Standard radiographs provide critical prognostic information for surgical repairs beyond the obvious need to exclude patients with glenohumeral arthritis. Decreased acromiohumeral interval (AHI) from superior humeral head migration not only correlates with the size of the tear but also with the stage of fatty degeneration of the muscle and portends worse outcomes [7–10]. Superior migration of the humeral head should be considered a contraindication to repair unless the tear is the result of acute trauma.

Rotator cuff fatty infiltration was initially described by Goutallier et al. [11] on arthro-CT imaging using a zero to four scale (Table 5.1). More recently, this classification was adapted to MRI. The pathogenesis of this change is a matter of debate. The prevailing theory suggests that mechanical unloading of the muscle increases the pennation angle of muscle fibers [12]. Interstitial

Table 5.1 Goutallier fatty degeneration staging

Stage 0	Completely normal muscle, no fatty streaks
Stage 1	Muscle contains some fatty streaks
Stage 2	More muscle than fat infiltration
Stage 3	Muscle equal to fat infiltration
Stage 4	More fat infiltration than muscle

fat and fibrous tissue fills in the spaces between the reoriented, retracted muscle fibers [13]. Increased connective tissue fibrosis, atrophy, and fatty infiltration all decrease the elasticity and viability of the rotator cuff. Increasing fatty infiltration and muscle atrophy have been correlated to higher re-tear rates after tendon repair [14–16] and are negative prognostic factors for clinical outcomes. Although the Goutallier zero to four scale is commonly used, a more simplified classification to better guide treatment would be to separate fatty infiltration into two groups. Patients with less fat than rotator cuff muscle are better candidates for repair than those patients in whom fat is present to an equal or greater extent than muscle. The latter can be considered tears that are unlikely to heal even if repair is technically possible. Gladstone and Flatow [17] have shown that advanced fatty atrophy seen preoperatively on an MRI did not reverse after surgical repair, even when tendon healing occurred, suggesting that muscle degeneration is permanent.

Treatment

The "healability" of a massive rotator cuff tear is a key consideration when determining the appropriate treatment. Other factors that play a role in treatment decisions include the patients' pain, function, as well as short- and long-term goals/expectations. Symptomatic patients below the age of 60 who have low levels of atrophy and fatty infiltration are ideal candidates for repair. Patients older than 60 should also be offered repair, but their age is a poor prognostic factor [18]. In patients with advanced atrophy or high-grade fatty infiltration, alternative treatments such as simple debridements, tendon transfers, or reverse arthroplasty should be considered.

Complete Repair: Posterosuperior Tears

Successful anatomic reconstruction of the rotator cuff leads to optimal short- and long-term outcomes as well as possibly decreased rates of arthropathy [19, 20], and complete repair of mas-

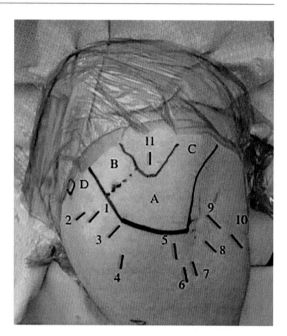

Fig. 5.1 The numerous possibilities for portal placement are shown. Recognition that the location of a portal is limited only by neurovascular structures frees the surgeon to establish portals as necessary to perform the repair. Most posterior-superior tears require a posterior portal (9), a lateral portal (6), and an anterior portal (2). Anchors can be placed percutaneously through small stab incisions lateral to the acromion. Subscapularis repair requires posterior (9), anterior (2), and accessory anterolateral (3) portals. Important bony landmarks and arthroscopic portals: (A) acromion, (B) clavicle, (C) scapular spine, (D) coracoid process. (1) anterosuperior portal, (2) anterior central portal, (3) superolateral portal, (4) anterolateral portal, (5) portal of Wilmington, (6) transrotator cuff portal, (7) posterolateral portal, (8) axillary pouch portal, (9) posterior portal, (10) 7 o'clock portal, (11) Neviaser portal

sive rotator cuff tears should be done whenever possible. The is little evidence to support the exclusive use of either the beach chair or lateral decubitus position, and setup should be done based on surgeon preference. A variety of portals facilitate this operation by allowing assessment of the torn tendon via different angles. Although many portals have been described, the surgeon should not feel constrained to only the use of these named portals. Ideal portal placement can be made at any location that does not risk injury to the neurovascular structures (Fig. 5.1).

Tension on a repaired tendon impairs tendon to bone healing [21]. Tendon retraction and scarring are common with chronic, massive tears and

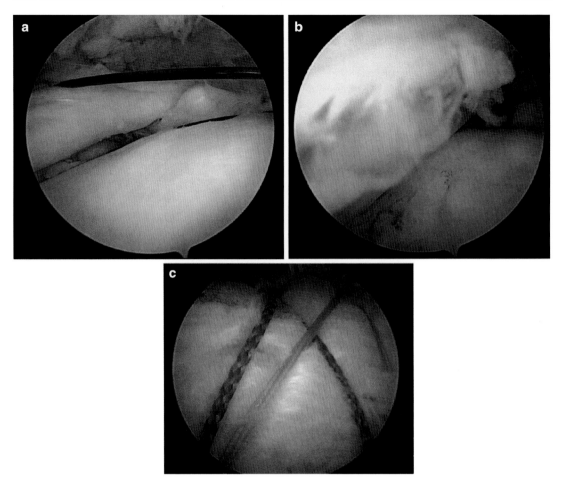

Fig. 5.2 (**a**) A traction stitch is placed at the apex of the retracted tear which exposes the humeral head. (**b**) The mobilized tear is lateralized to the tuberosity with a gentle pull on the traction stitch. This technique aids in releasing tendon adhesions and with suture passing. (**c**) A double-row repair compresses the tendon to the footprint, increasing contact area for healing

must be addressed to achieve adequate mobilization for a successful repair. Mobilization is critical not only for repair but also to free the muscle-tendon units to freely glide for motion.

A stepwise method of releasing the scarred and medialized tendons can be used and is greatly facilitated by the use of traction stitches (Fig. 5.2). The principles of this method are the same as with open repair. Traction stitches are placed at the apex of the tear and externalized through small mini-portals placed to create an optimal vector for tear reduction. Tendon excursion can first be increased by release of all bursal-sided adhesions, both subacromial and subdeltoid [22]. This is best done by viewing through a lateral or posterolateral portal and dissecting in the plane immediately above the rotator cuff.

If bursal-sided releases do not produce sufficient excursion, articular-sided adhesions are then addressed. With chronic retracted tendon tears, the tendon and capsule may become scarred to the glenoid rim and must be released (Fig. 5.3). This can safely be performed by starting at the rotator interval and working posteriorly [23]. Dissection should not extend more than 2 cm past the glenoid neck in order to avoid suprascapular nerve injury.

If the above techniques do not afford sufficient mobility and there is differential retraction of adjacent tendons, interval slides can be performed.

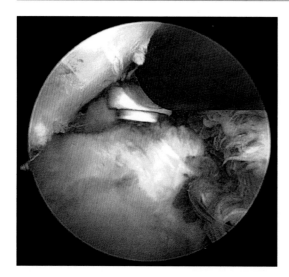

Fig. 5.3 Articular-sided releases are performed by dissecting between the rotator cuff and the superior labrum to release capsular adhesions. Looking from the lateral portal, the electrocautery is slid under the cuff and the capsule is released. The glenoid is seen inferiorly. The dissection should not extend more than 2 cm medially to avoid suprascapular nerve injury. Traction on the cuff during this release aids in identifying sites of adhesion

These arthroscopic techniques are modifications to those originally performed during open surgery. If the supraspinatus is retracted and scarred to an intact subscapularis, the arthroscopic anterior slide is performed by releasing the interval between the subscapularis and supraspinatus tendons [24, 25]. The coracohumeral ligament, which has often become contracted and tethered, is also incised off of the coracoid process.

The posterior interval slide can provide additional tendon excursion if there is unequal retraction of the supraspinatus and infraspinatus. This release is performed between the two adjacent musculotendinous units [26]. The scapular spine can be delineated by removing excess subacromial fibroadipose tissue. This anatomical landmark serves as the boundary between the two units and directs the accurate release of the interval between them. The posterior interval slide allows increased excursion of both muscle units.

Collectively, double-interval slides can afford over 5 cm of mobility to the posterosuperior rotator cuff. However, because suprascapular nerve injuries have been reported with greater than 3 cm of mobility, surgeons should be cautious with over-mobilization [27].

Some massive rotator cuffs can be further mobilized with utilization of margin convergence. Though initially described by Inman [28], Burkhart coined the term to describe a side-to-side closure of the anterior and posterior tendon leafs [29]. Traditionally, U-shaped tears were closed by mobilizing the medial, retracted margin back to its bony bed. This technique resulted in high tensile stresses that predisposed to eventual repair failure. The technique of margin convergence utilizes sequential tendon sutures, starting medially and working laterally, causing the free margin of the tear to converge toward its bone bed, offloading the strain on the repair and leaving a tension-free cuff margin to be repaired to the footprint (Fig. 5.4). The biomechanical benefits of margin convergence have been borne out in several studies, with side-to-side repair of two-thirds of a U-shaped tear resulting in one-sixth the strain across the repair site. Mazzocca [30] showed in an open cadaveric study that margin convergence also has a significant role for large retracted rotator cuff tears, with sequential side-to-side sutures resulting in progressive gap closure as well as decreased repair strain.

The optimal technique for reattachment of the tendon to the bone has been widely researched, but no consensus has been reached yet. Gerber et al. [31] described the characteristics of the optimal rotator cuff repair as having (1) high initial fixation strength, (2) minimal gap formation, and (3) sustained mechanical stability until healing has occurred. Some factors analyzed to enhance repair constructs include utilization of stronger suture, various methods of knot tying, and analysis of anchor fixation biomechanics. Recently, much interest has focused on the results of single-/double-row repairs and transosseous equivalent repairs. Double-row fixation has been shown to have improved initial strength and stiffness and decreased gap formation compared with single-row repairs [32]. In a cadaveric study by Brady et al. [33], more than half of the anatomic footprint remained uncovered with single-row fixation, whereas near complete coverage was gained with double-row fixation. The transosseous equivalent

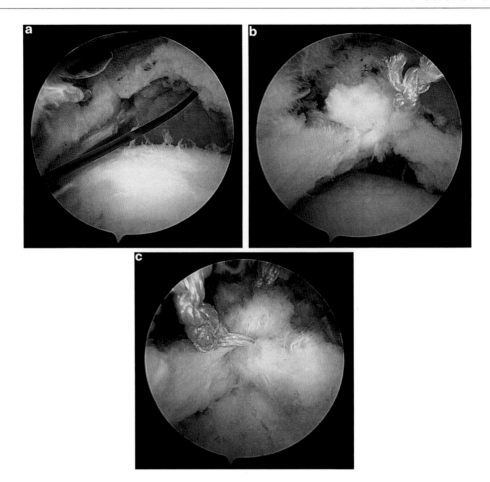

Fig. 5.4 The technique of marginal convergence can be used to address a "U"- or "V"-shaped tear. (**a**) A "V"-shaped tear seen from a lateral portal. (**b**) Sutures passed anteriorly to posteriorly closing the V and converging the lateral edge of the tendon to the tuberosity. (**c**) The lateral edge is brought to the footprint under little tension

technique utilizes a medial row of suture anchors placed lateral to the articular surface, with crossing sutures to a lateral row of suture anchors placed in the greater tuberosity. This technique compresses the free edge of the rotator cuff tendon down onto its footprint, thereby increasing surface area contact for tendon to bone healing (Fig. 5.2c). Transosseous equivalent repairs better recreate the native footprint of the cuff compared with single- and double-row repairs and improve contact area for healing.

Despite these theoretical structural benefits, most studies have not shown a clinical benefit to double-row repairs when analyzing arthroscopic tendon repairs of all tear sizes. Park et al. [34] stratified patients by tear size and found that large or massive rotator cuff tears (>3 cm) had significantly improved function with double-row fixation, suggesting that this technique may be more suitable for larger tears. Careful consideration should be made when using double-row fixation particularly in massive rotator cuff tears since over-tensioning of the repair is potentially higher in these cases (as compared with smaller tears). Since few studies have investigated this issue in massive rotator cuff tears, additional research must be done to further assess for any potential clinical benefits and to define the circumstances for the utilization of either technique.

Outcomes

Re-tear rates after arthroscopic repair of massive rotator cuff tears are relatively high, ranging from 25 to 90 % [1, 35, 36]. Despite these high rates of healing failure, functional outcomes and satisfaction rates have only been marginally associated with tendon healing success and, instead, have consistently been shown to be favorable.

Yoo et al. [37] reported on 89 patients with large to massive rotator cuff tears repaired arthroscopically. At a mean follow-up of 30 months, they found a re-tear rate of 45.5 % but with significantly improved pain and function scores. No difference was noted between re-tear and non-re-tear groups. Similar findings were reported by Chung et al. [19], who studied 108 arthroscopically repaired massive rotator cuffs. At a mean follow-up of 32 months, they found 40 % of patients had a recurrence of their tear, though the mean defect size was significantly smaller than the initial tear size. All functional outcome scores significantly improved and were not significantly different between healed and unhealed cuffs. They also noted that degree of fatty infiltration significantly predisposed to healing failure in a multivariate analysis.

Longer follow-up studies confirm durability of functional outcome improvements. Galatz et al. [1] studied outcomes in 18 patients who had arthroscopic repairs of tears >2 cm in the transverse plane, with mean follow-up of 36 months. Recurrent tears were seen in 17 of the 18 patients as measured using ultrasound, with many tears measuring the same size as before surgery. Nevertheless, 13 patients had American Shoulder and Elbow Surgeons (ASES) scores >90 points at 1 year, with significant improvement in pain relief, range of motion, strength, and ability to perform activities of daily living. By 2-year follow-up, the average ASES score declined to 80. A 10-year follow-up study [38] of the same cohort of patients with re-torn rotator cuffs showed unchanged ASES and pain scores, though all patients had evidence of degenerative radiographic changes. The authors concluded that healing of the rotator cuff was not vital for successful outcome of tear repairs and that early *clinical* improvement was durable at long-term follow-up.

Anterosuperior Rotator Cuff Repair

In the past, anterosuperior tears were less commonly diagnosed and treated, likely because they were not diagnosed [1, 31, 39]. Improved methods of clinical and radiographic evaluation, as well as the widespread use of arthroscopy, have led to increased recognition and an improved understanding of their significance [40–42]. Arthroscopic treatment of these tears has lagged behind that of other rotator cuff pathology because it is technically difficult, and there is potential for injury to the neurovascular structures which are in close proximity to a medially retracted tendon. Promising results with arthroscopic repairs have been reported, however [40, 43–46]. The subscapularis is an integral part of the anterior-posterior force couple which maintains ball and socket kinematics during humeral abduction [47], and rotator cuff tears which involve the subscapularis have inferior outcomes following repair compared with those that do not [48].

Arthroscopic treatment of anterosuperior tears generally can be performed through three working portals. Due to the retroversion of the humeral neck, the anterior deltoid muscle naturally drapes over the footprint of the subscapularis tendon and limits visualization during the repair. With increased operative time, swelling from fluid extravasation can exacerbate this problem [49]. After general diagnostic arthroscopy, the subscapularis tendon is repaired before the biceps or any of the other rotator cuff tendons.

Identification of the tendon edge may be difficult, depending the severity of muscle retraction (Fig. 5.5). The inferior muscular portion of the subscapularis may be intact and attached to the lesser tuberosity [49]. In these cases, this retained segment can be followed proximally to the retracted tendinous portion. Recognition of the tendon can also be identified by the "comma sign," a structure formed by parts of the superior glenohumeral ligament and the coracohumeral

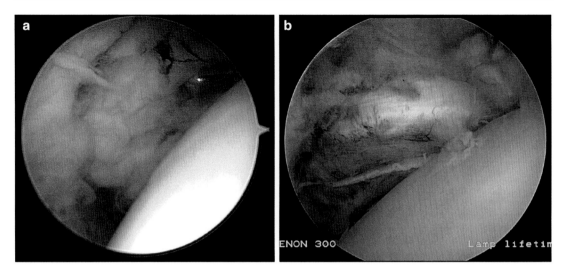

Fig. 5.5 In contrast to superior and posterior tears, tears of the subscapularis rarely appear as a discrete hole at the time of arthroscopy. With careful examination of the anterior joint, the superior "rolled" edge of the tendon should be identified. If it is not obviously seen and a tear is present, the surgeon should look medially for a retracted tendon. (**a**) Shows the view from the posterior portal of a torn subscapularis. (**b**) Demonstrates the restoration of the superior rolled edge after repair

ligament that is consistently located along the superolateral aspect of the tendon [6, 40]. During tearing of the tendon, this complex avulses off of the humerus along with the medial sling of the biceps tendon.

The retracted tendon is often scarred and tethered, and circumferential releases should be performed. The releases done arthroscopically mimicked those used in open surgery. The superior edge is freed from rotator interval tissue and from adhesions to the coracoid. Again, mobilization is aided by the use of traction sutures placed through the tendon edge and externalized through percutaneous mini-portals made so that the vector of the traction stitch draws the tendon to its anatomic location. The subscapularis tendon is then released from the anterior joint capsule and freed of adhesions in the subcoracoid space, as needed. If dissection below the inferior half of the tendon is required, the axillary nerve is identified and protected. This is best done by blunt dissection anteromedially in the subcoracoid space. The comma is preserved when the tear includes the supraspinatus (Fig. 5.6). Coracoplasty may also be required in select cases. A burr is used to resect the lateral tip and posterior aspect of the

coracoid to widen the coracohumeral window for the subscapularis tendon [49]. Narrow windows have been associated with increased subscapularis tear rates.

An outside-in technique for passing sutures is a safe and effective method of repair. Viewing intra-articularly from the posterior portal, sutures from anchors in the lesser tuberosity are laid posteriorly to the subscapularis tendon. A pointed grasper is then used to pierce the subscapularis tendon from the superficial through the deep surface of the tendon to grasp the suture. It is then pulled back through the tendon and tied in the subdeltoid space. This is repeated for each suture starting from the most distal and moving proximally. Once the subscapularis tendon has been repaired, attention can be turned to the supraspinatus/infraspinatus repairs as needed. Biceps pathology should also be addressed with either tenodesis or tenotomy.

Outcomes

Studies looking at arthroscopic anterosuperior tear repair are relatively sparse, but all have shown significant benefits for affected patients.

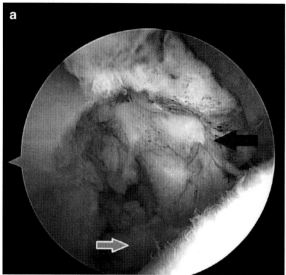
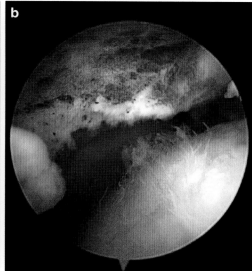

Fig. 5.6 (a) Preservation of the comma tissue (*red arrow*) connecting the subscapularis (*blue arrow*) and the supraspinatus can reduce strain on the repair and aid in reducing the supraspinatus. (b) After the subscapularis is repaired, the preserved comma lateralizes the supraspinatus toward the tuberosity

Burkhart et al. [40] retrospectively studied 25 cases of subscapularis tendon tears, with 17 involving the supraspinatus or infraspinatus tendons. At a mean of 10.7 months, UCLA function scores improved significantly.

Ide et al. [49] performed a prospective study on 20 patients arthroscopically treated for anterosuperior tendon tears, with 7 patients having infraspinatus tendon extension. At 36 months' follow-up, 13 of 20 patients had intact repairs as identified by MRI. All patients were found to have improved outcome scores, though patients with re-tears had less improvement than those that had intact repairs. Older age and degree of retraction correlated with re-tearing of the tendon.

Nho et al. [50] most recently analyzed outcomes in 13 patients who underwent arthroscopic repair of anterosuperior tears. Coracoplasties and open biceps tenodeses were performed on all patients. At final mean follow-up of 35 months, all patients showed significant improvement in ASES outcome scores, with eleven noting that they were "delighted" by their outcome.

Rehabilitation

Rehabilitation after open rotator cuff repairs has traditionally been instituted early to prevent postoperative stiffness due to subdeltoid adhesions. The minimal trauma from arthroscopy has been associated a lower incidence of stiffness [51], and the growing concern over high re-tear rates has prompted investigation into delayed rehabilitation. Parsons et al. [52] evaluated 43 patients with full-thickness rotator cuff repairs who underwent sling immobilization without therapy for 6 weeks. Though 23 % of patients became "stiff" at the 6–8-week follow-up, range of motion was similar at 1-year follow-up between stiff and non-stiff groups after physical therapy, and healing rates improved in the delayed therapy group. For this reason, it is the author's practice to keep patients with massive rotator cuff repairs immobilized in a sling at all times for 6 weeks, in order to optimize tendon to bone healing. Gentle therapy can be started after this time with a focus on regaining motion and smooth scapulohumeral rhythm. Strengthening is not begun until 4 months after surgery and is rarely emphasized.

Partial Repair

Although mobilization of the rotator cuff can be done through release of adhesions and interval slides, atrophy and poor tissue quality may prevent complete repair of the torn tendon to its anatomic footprint. In these cases, partial repair may be considered. Though it may have less favorable outcomes when compared with complete repairs, adequate function can be restored and predictable pain relief achieved. This technique may be best suited for patients who have an acute decline in function following an injury and are found to have preexisting irreparable tears. In this situation, it is reasonable to complete a partial repair in an attempt to restore their preinjury level of function.

The "functional rotator cuff tear" concept led to the rationale behind partial repairs. Restoration of the anterior and posterior humeral head depressors creates a fixed fulcrum for the deltoid lever. Repair of the infraspinatus alone in posterior-superior tears (or the subscapularis in anterosuperior tears) often restores function and range of motion, despite the residual defect in the repair. It is important to understand that creating this stable fulcrum for motion is more important than anatomically closing the deficiency of the tear. Utilization of margin convergence, in combination, further enhances the repair by decreasing strain on the fixation.

Outcomes

Several studies have supported this technique, with good functional results. Duralde et al. [39] showed 24 cases in which complete repair was not possible. Open partial repairs of massive rotator cuff tears showed an improvement in forward elevation from 114° preoperatively to 154° postoperatively, and 92 % of patients were satisfied with their result. Similarly, in his group of open

repairs, Burkhart et al. [53] showed a gain of 90° in forward elevation and increased UCLA scores from 10 to 28. In a study by Berth et al. [54], both arthroscopic partial repairs and arthroscopic debridements showed significant decreases in pain and improvement in function, with partial repairs resulting in greater improvement in shoulder function.

Iagulli et al. [55] compared results from arthroscopic partial and complete rotator cuff repairs. In this series of 97 patients, 54 % achieved a complete repair, whereas 46 % underwent partial repair. Both groups showed significant improvements in UCLA scores and function. Interestingly, satisfaction rates between the two groups were comparable, and outcomes were not significantly different between the two groups. The authors suggest that partial repair of massive rotator cuff tears can yield results equivalent to complete repair in short-term follow-up. Further studies may need to be performed to assess the durability of these results.

Irreparable Tears

When repair is not possible, additional arthroscopic options exist for treatment of massive rotator cuff tears, including subacromial decompression, biceps tenodesis/tenotomy, and management of suprascapular neuropathy. Though strength may not improve with these modalities, pain relief is often an achievable goal.

Long Head of the Biceps Tendon

Tendinopathy of the long head of the biceps (LHB) is associated with massive rotator cuff tears and frequently causes pain. In patients with massive rotator cuff tears, LHB pathology ranges from structural tearing and delamination to frank subluxation and dislocation. Isolated biceps tenotomy or tenodesis is an attractive option for low-demand patients with irreparable tears or those patients that are unwilling or unable to participate in postoperative rehabilitation. This procedure affords reliable pain relief with minimal recovery time.

Outcomes

Walch et al. [56] reported on 307 patients who underwent arthroscopic biceps tenotomies for full-thickness rotator cuff tears. All had irreparable tears or were unwilling to participate in the required rehabilitation after a rotator cuff repair. Over 66 % of rotator cuff tears involved at least 2 tendons. At an average of 57-month follow-up, mean Constant scores significantly improved, and 87 % of patients were satisfied with their result. Evidence of glenohumeral arthritis increased from 38 to 67 %, suggesting that tenotomies do not slow progression of radiographic changes, but only 2 % of patients in this study went on to reverse shoulder arthroplasty. Kempf et al. [57] found similar results with LHB tenotomy, concluding in their multicenter study that LHB tenotomy was particularly effective in patients with massive rotator cuff tears.

Boileau et al. [58] also investigated the results of biceps tendon management for massive rotator cuff tears with comparisons between tenodesis and tenotomy. Both modalities were successful, with an overall satisfaction rating over 78 % and significant improvements in Constant scores. Patients with pseudoparalysis, though, did not regain functional arm elevation and therefore would not be good candidates for this procedure. Outcome scores were similar between tenodesis and tenotomy, though tenotomies had higher rates of cosmetic deformity.

Suprascapular Neuropathy

There is a growing body of evidence that rotator cuff tears are associated with significant suprascapular nerve dysfunction. Anatomically, the suprascapular nerve arises from the brachial plexus and passes underneath the transverse scapular ligament to innervate the supraspinatus and infraspinatus. It has contributions from the nerve roots of C5 and C6 and variable contributions from C4. Massive rotator cuff tears that have retracted may produce excessive traction on the nerve due to a tethering effect on it at its relatively immobile position beneath the transverse scapular ligament. Warner and colleagues [59] found that suprascapular neuropathy noted on electromyography and nerve conduction studies did not correlate to fatty infiltration found on MRI. Cadaveric studies have verified increased tension on the nerve with supraspinatus retraction, resulting from a decreased angle between the suprascapular nerve and its first motor branch [60]. Mallon et al. [61] reported a series of 8 patients with massive rotator cuff tears that all had EMG findings consistent with suprascapular neuropathy. Fortunately, this stretch injury may be reversed with repair of the tear; both patients who had follow-up EMGs following partial rotator cuff repairs for massive tears had significant re-innervation potentials. Costouros et al. [62] found similar results in his study of 7 patients with massive rotator cuff tears and isolated suprascapular neuropathy treated with arthroscopic partial or complete repair. In their EMG follow-up of 6 patients, all had partial or full recovery of nerve function with associated pain relief and functional improvement. Whether there is a role for releasing the suprascapular nerve in tears that cannot be repaired remains a matter of debate.

Conclusion

Massive rotator cuff tears can be severely debilitating and present a challenging problem. Arthroscopic techniques have several advantages over traditional open repairs and technological advances have greatly improved the arthroscopic management. Biologic considerations dictate the appropriate treatment in most cases, and anatomic repair remains the ideal treatment when possible. Partial repair can also restore function and provide pain relief. The many options for irreparable tendon tears include debridement, biceps tenodesis/tenotomy, and salvage procedures discussed elsewhere in this book. The role of suprascapular nerve decompression remains undefined but may prove valuable in the setting of a retracted, irreparable tear.

References

1. Galatz LM, Ball CM, Teefey SA, Middleton WD, Yamaguchi K. The outcome and repair integrity of completely arthroscopically repaired large and massive rotator cuff tears. J Bone Joint Surg Am. 2004;86-A:219–24.
2. Cofield RH, Parvizi J, Hoffmeyer PJ, Lanzer WL, Ilstrup DM, Rowland CM. Surgical repair of chronic rotator cuff tears. A prospective long-term study. J Bone Joint Surg Am. 2001;83-A:71–7.
3. Burkhart SS. Arthroscopic treatment of massive rotator cuff tears. Clinical results and biomechanical rationale. Clin Orthop Relat Res. 1991;267:45–56.
4. Zumstein MA, Jost B, Hempel J, Hodler J, Gerber C. The clinical and structural long-term results of open repair of massive tears of the rotator cuff. J Bone Joint Surg Am. 2008;90:2423–31.
5. Harryman 2nd DT, Hettrich CM, Smith KL, Campbell B, Sidles JA, Matsen 3rd FA. A prospective multipractice investigation of patients with full-thickness rotator cuff tears: the importance of comorbidities. Practice, and other covariables on self-assessed shoulder function and health status. J Bone Joint Surg Am. 2003;85-A:690–6.
6. Burkhart SS, Lo IK. Arthroscopic rotator cuff repair. J Am Acad Orthop Surg. 2006;14:333–46.
7. Ellman H, Hanker G, Bayer M. Repair of the rotator cuff. End-result study of factors influencing reconstruction. J Bone Joint Surg Am. 1986;68:1136–44.
8. Hamada K, Fukuda H, Mikasa M, Kobayashi Y. Roentgenographic findings in massive rotator cuff tears. A long-term observation. Clin Orthop Relat Res. 1990;254:92–6.
9. Vad VB, Warren RF, Altchek DW, O'Brien SJ, Rose HA, Wickiewicz TL. Negative prognostic factors in managing massive rotator cuff tears. Clin J Sport Med. 2002;12:151–7.
10. Werner CM, Conrad SJ, Meyer DC, Keller A, Hodler J, Gerber C. Intermethod agreement and interobserver correlation of radiologic acromiohumeral distance measurements. J Shoulder Elbow Surg. 2008;17:237–40.
11. Goutallier D, Postel JM, Bernageau J, Lavau L, Voisin MC. Fatty muscle degeneration in cuff ruptures. Pre- and postoperative evaluation by CT scan. Clin Orthop Relat Res. 1994;304:78–83.
12. Tomioka T, Minagawa H, Kijima H, Yamamoto N, Abe H, Maesani M, et al. Sarcomere length of torn rotator cuff muscle. J Shoulder Elbow Surg. 2009;18:955–9.
13. Kuzel BR, Grindel S, Papandrea R, Ziegler D. Fatty infiltration and rotator cuff atrophy. J Am Acad Orthop Surg. 2013;21:613–23.
14. Gerber C, Fuchs B, Hodler J. The results of repair of massive tears of the rotator cuff. J Bone Joint Surg Am. 2000;82:505–15.
15. Goutallier D, Postel JM, Gleyze P, Leguilloux P, Van Driessche S. Influence of cuff muscle fatty degeneration on anatomic and functional outcomes after simple suture of full-thickness tears. J Shoulder Elbow Surg. 2003;12:550–4.
16. Mellado JM, Calmet J, Olona M, Esteve C, Camins A, Perez Del Palomar L, et al. Surgically repaired massive rotator cuff tears: MRI of tendon integrity. Muscle fatty degeneration, and muscle atrophy correlated with intraoperative and clinical findings. AJR Am J Roentgenol. 2005;184:1456–63.
17. Gladstone JN, Bishop JY, Lo IK, Flatow EL. Fatty infiltration and atrophy of the rotator cuff do not improve after rotator cuff repair and correlate with poor functional outcome. Am J Sports Med. 2007;35:719–28.
18. Tashjian RZ, Hollins AM, Kim HM, Teefey SA, Middleton WD, Steger-May K, et al. Factors affecting healing rates after arthroscopic double-row rotator cuff repair. Am J Sports Med. 2010;38:2435–42.
19. Chung SW, Kim JY, Kim MH, Kim SH, Oh JH. Arthroscopic repair of massive rotator cuff tears: outcome and analysis of factors associated with healing failure or poor postoperative function, Am J Sports Med. 2013;41:1674–83.
20. Kim KC, Shin HD, Lee WY. Repair integrity and functional outcomes after arthroscopic suture-bridge rotator cuff repair. J Bone Joint Surg Am. 2012;94:e48.
21. Gimbel JA, Van Kleunen JP, Lake SP, Williams GR, Soslowsky LJ. The role of repair tension on tendon to bone healing in an animal model of chronic rotator cuff tears. J Biomech. 2007;40:561–8.
22. Bedi A, Dines J, Warren RF, Dines DM. Massive tears of the rotator cuff. J Bone Joint Surg Am. 2010; 92:1894–908.
23. Neri BR, Chan KW, Kwon YW. Management of massive and irreparable rotator cuff tears. J Shoulder Elbow Surg. 2009;18:808–18.
24. Cordasco FA, Bigliani LU. The rotator cuff. Large and massive tears. Technique of open repair. Orthop Clin North Am. 1997;28:179–93.
25. Tauro JC. Arthroscopic "interval slide" in the repair of large rotator cuff tears. Arthroscopy. 1999;15:527–30.
26. Lo IK, Burkhart SS. Arthroscopic repair of massive, contracted, immobile rotator cuff tears using single and double interval slides: technique and preliminary results. Arthroscopy. 2004;20:22–33.
27. Hoellrich RG, Gasser SI, Morrison DS, Kurzweil PR. Electromyographic evaluation after primary repair of massive rotator cuff tears. J Shoulder Elbow Surg. 2005;14:269–72.
28. Inman VT, Saunders JB, Abbott LC. Observations of the function of the shoulder joint. 1944. Clin Orthop Relat Res. 1996;330:3–12.
29. Burkhart SS, Athanasiou KA, Wirth MA. Margin convergence: a method of reducing strain in massive rotator cuff tears. Arthroscopy. 1996;12:335–8.
30. Mazzocca AD, Bollier M, Fehsenfeld D, Romeo A, Stephens K, Solovyoya O, et al. Biomechanical evalu-

ation of margin convergence. Arthroscopy. 2011; 27:330–8.

31. Gerber C, Schneeberger AG, Beck M, Schlegel U. Mechanical strength of repairs of the rotator cuff. J Bone Joint Surg Br. 1994;76:371–80.

32. Kim DH, Elattrache NS, Tibone JE, Jun BJ, DeLaMora SN, Kvitne RS, et al. Biomechanical comparison of a single-row versus double-row suture anchor technique for rotator cuff repair. Am J Sports Med. 2006;34:407–14.

33. Brady PC, Arrigoni P, Burkhart SS. Evaluation of residual rotator cuff defects after in vivo single- versus double-row rotator cuff repairs. Arthroscopy. 2006;22:1070–5.

34. Park JY, Lhee SH, Choi JH, Park HK, Yu JW, Seo JB. Comparison of the clinical outcomes of single- and double-row repairs in rotator cuff tears. Am J Sports Med. 2008;36:1310–6.

35. Boileau P, Brassart N, Watkinson DJ, Carles M, Hatzidakis AM, Krishnan SG. Arthroscopic repair of full-thickness tears of the supraspinatus: does the tendon really heal? J Bone Joint Surg Am. 2005;87:1229–40.

36. Park JY, Lhee SH, Oh KS, Moon SG, Hwang JT. Clinical and ultrasonographic outcomes of arthroscopic suture bridge repair for massive rotator cuff tear. Arthroscopy. 2013;29:280–9.

37. Yoo JC, Ahn JH, Koh KH, Lim KS. Rotator cuff integrity after arthroscopic repair for large tears with less-than-optimal footprint coverage. Arthroscopy. 2009;25:1093–100.

38. Paxton ES, Teefey SA, Dahiya N, Keener JD, Yamaguchi K, Galatz LM. Clinical and radiographic outcomes of failed repairs of large or massive rotator cuff tears: minimum ten-year follow-up. J Bone Joint Surg Am. 2013;95:627–32.

39. Duralde XA, Bair B. Massive rotator cuff tears: the result of partial rotator cuff repair. J Shoulder Elbow Surg. 2005;14:121–7.

40. Burkhart SS, Tehrany AM. Arthroscopic subscapularis tendon repair: technique and preliminary results. Arthroscopy. 2002;18:454–63.

41. Gerber C, Krushell RJ. Isolated rupture of the tendon of the subscapularis muscle. Clinical features in 16 cases. J Bone Joint Surg Br. 1991;73:389–94.

42. Pfirrmann CW, Zanetti M, Weishaupt D, Gerber C, Hodler J. Subscapularis tendon tears: detection and grading at MR arthrography. Radiology. 1999;213: 709–14.

43. Adams CR, Schoolfield JD, Burkhart SS. The results of arthroscopic subscapularis tendon repairs. Arthroscopy. 2008;24:1381–9.

44. Arai R, Sugaya H, Mochizuki T, Nimura A, Moriishi J, Akita K. Subscapularis tendon tear: an anatomic and clinical investigation. Arthroscopy. 2008;24: 997–1004.

45. Bartl C, Salzmann GM, Seppel G, Eichhorn S, Holzapfel K, Wortler K, et al. Subscapularis function and structural integrity after arthroscopic repair of isolated subscapularis tears. Am J Sports Med. 2011;39:1255–62.

46. Lafosse L, Jost B, Reiland Y, Audebert S, Toussaint B, Gobezie R. Structural integrity and clinical outcomes after arthroscopic repair of isolated subscapularis tears. J Bone Joint Surg Am. 2007;89:1184–93.

47. Thompson WO, Debski RE, Boardman 3rd ND, Taskiran E, Warner JJ, Fu FH, et al. A biomechanical analysis of rotator cuff deficiency in a cadaveric model. Am J Sports Med. 1996;24:286–92.

48. Millett PJ, Horan MP, Maland KE, Hawkins RJ. Long-term survivorship and outcomes after surgical repair of full-thickness rotator cuff tears. J Shoulder Elbow Surg. 2011;20:591–7.

49. Ide J, Tokiyoshi A, Hirose J, Mizuta H. Arthroscopic repair of traumatic combined rotator cuff tears involving the subscapularis tendon. J Bone Joint Surg Am. 2007;89:2378–88.

50. Nho SJ, Frank RM, Reiff SN, Verma NN, Romeo AA. Arthroscopic repair of anterosuperior rotator cuff tears combined with open biceps tenodesis. Arthroscopy. 2010;26:1667–74.

51. Brislin KJ, Field LD, Savoie 3rd FH. Complications after arthroscopic rotator cuff repair. Arthroscopy. 2007;23:124–8.

52. Parsons BO, Gruson KI, Chen DD, Harrison AK, Gladstone J, Flatow EL. Does slower rehabilitation after arthroscopic rotator cuff repair lead to long-term stiffness? J Shoulder Elbow Surg. 2010; 19:1034–9.

53. Burkhart SS, Nottage WM, Ogilvie-Harris DJ, Kohn HS, Pachelli A. Partial repair of irreparable rotator cuff tears. Arthroscopy. 1994;10:363–70.

54. Berth A, Neumann W, Awiszus F, Pap G. Massive rotator cuff tears: functional outcome after debridement or arthroscopic partial repair. J Orthop Traumatol. 2010;11:13–20.

55. Iagulli ND, Field LD, Hobgood ER, Ramsey JR, Savoie 3rd FH. Comparison of partial versus complete arthroscopic repair of massive rotator cuff tears. Am J Sports Med. 2012;40:1022–6.

56. Walch G, Edwards TB, Boulahia A, Nove-Josserand L, Neyton L, Szabo I. Arthroscopic tenotomy of the long head of the biceps in the treatment of rotator cuff tears: clinical and radiographic results of 307 cases. J Shoulder Elbow Surg. 2005;14:238–46.

57. Kempf JF, Gleyze P, Bonnomet F, Walch G, Mole D, Frank A, et al. A multicenter study of 210 rotator cuff tears treated by arthroscopic acromioplasty. Arthroscopy. 1999;15:56–66.

58. Boileau P, Baque F, Valerio L, Ahrens P, Chuinard C, Trojani C. Isolated arthroscopic biceps tenotomy or tenodesis improves symptoms in patients with massive irreparable rotator cuff tears. J Bone Joint Surg Am. 2007;89:747–57.

59. Shi LL, Boykin RE, Lin A, Warner JJ. Association of suprascapular neuropathy with rotator cuff tendon tears and fatty degeneration. J Shoulder Elbow Surg. 2014;23:339–46.

60. Albritton MJ, Graham RD, Richards 2nd RS, Basamania CJ. An anatomic study of the effects on the suprascapular nerve due to retraction of the supra-

spinatus muscle after a rotator cuff tear. J Shoulder Elbow Surg. 2003;12:497–500.

61. Mallon WJ, Wilson RJ, Basamania CJ. The association of suprascapular neuropathy with massive rotator cuff tears: a preliminary report. J Shoulder Elbow Surg. 2006;15:395–8.

62. Costouros JG, Porramatikul M, Lie DT, Warner JJ. Reversal of suprascapular neuropathy following arthroscopic repair of massive supraspinatus and infraspinatus rotator cuff tears. Arthroscopy. 2007; 23:1152–61.

Biologics and Patches

6

Phillip N. Williams, Jaydev B. Mistry, and Joshua S. Dines

P.N. Williams, MD
Department of Orthopaedic Surgery,
Hospital for Special Surgery,
535 E 70th Street, New York, NY 10021, USA
e-mail: WilliamsP@hss.edu

J.B. Mistry, BA
Rutgers New Jersey Medical School,
Medical Sciences Building, 185 South
Orange Ave, Newark, NJ 07103, USA
e-mail: mistryjb@njms.rutgers.edu

J.S. Dines, MD (⊠)
Sports Medicine and Shoulder Service,
Hospital for Special Surgery, New York, NY, USA

Department of Orthopaedic Surgery,
Weill Cornell Medical College, New York, NY, USA
e-mail: jdinesmd@gmail.com

Pearls and Pitfalls

Pearls

- Future research should focus on ways to biologically augment rotator cuff tears in order to reduce retear rates and increase healing rates.
- Patches may be used to augment the repair of massive rotator cuff tears in the setting of compromised tissue quality, revision surgery, and in those patients with medical issues that may predispose them to poor healing (i.e., diabetes)
- Transosseous-equivalent, double-row rotator cuff repairs may facilitate arthroscopic insertion of patches.
- After the medial row sutures have been tied, the suture ends can be sutured through the patch and then shuttled down the cannula. The free sutures can then be secured to lateral knotless anchors in order to secure the patch.

Pitfalls

- There is insufficient evidence to support the routine use of PRP to augment rotator cuff repairs.
- Porcine small intestine submucosa should not be used for rotator cuff repair augmentation.
- Grafts should not be used for interposition, but rather for tissue augmentation.
- Open or mini-open repairs can be performed with patches until comfort is achieved with arthroscopic placement and fixation.

Introduction

More than 150,000 rotator cuff repair operations are performed annually in the United States. While the overwhelming majority of patients will do well after the procedure, there is a subset of patients who continue to experience pain and functional disability [1, 2]. In many of these cases, the inferior outcomes are directly attributable to either (a) the repaired tendon failing to heal or (b) retearing. Retear (or failure to heal) rates have been reported to range from 10 % in smaller tears to 90 % in massive tears [3, 4]. Higher failure rates are found in larger tears and poor-quality tendons, which can be partly attributed to chronic disease, fatty infiltration of muscle fibers, and muscle atrophy. Tendons typically heal through reactive scar tissue formation that is mechanically weaker than native tendon.

Over the past decade, surgical instrumentation and repair constructs have improved significantly, decreasing mechanical failure as the reason tendons fail to heal. Several repair constructs, such as double-row and transosseous-equivalent repairs, not only improve the biomechanical strength of the repaired tendon but also provide better biological environments for healing. Moving forward, it will clearly be our ability to manipulate the biologic milieu of the healing tendon that will provide improved outcomes to our patients.

At this point, much of the research focusing on enhancing tendon healing is in the preclinical stages. They will be reviewed here, but the focus of the chapter will be on modalities available to surgeons now including platelet rich plasma (PRP) and patches. It is important to note that patient selection is a critical element of improving outcomes. While beyond the scope of this chapter, optimizing the medical condition of patients with massive tears via better medical management of diabetics and smokers may be the most effective way to currently improve the biology of the healing environment (see Pearls and Pitfalls).

Platelet Rich Plasma (PRP)

Cytokines such as PDGF-β, TGF-β, BMPs, IGF-1, VEGF, and FGF play documented roles in the healing process. Cell proliferation, matrix synthesis, and angiogenesis are all fundamental processes affected by cytokines. Improving these processes would potentially increase the body's ability to heal a tendon repair via the normal tendon enthesis, as opposed to scar tissue.

PRP is, by definition, a sample of autologous blood with a platelet concentration of at least 3× the baseline. The concentration of platelets exploits the fact that α-granules of platelets contain the abovementioned cytokines and growth factors critical to the healing process. However, the concentration of cytokines and growth factors released is variable and depends upon the platelet recovery method, amount of whole blood used, platelet activation, final volume of platelets, and other variables. Additionally, the formulation of PRP, liquid versus solid, plays an important role in determining its bioavailability. While, the liquid form allows injection into the area of the rotator cuff repair, it only remains for 7–12 h. Whereas the solid form allows elution of growth factors for up to 7 days. However, the later must be sutured into the interface between the tendon and bone and can pose technical challenges [5].

Although PRP holds much promise for healing, clinical data has been difficult to interpret because of inconsistent and sometimes contradictory results. Castricini et al. [6] randomized 88 patients undergoing rotator cuff repair with and without a single PRP matrix globule and used the constant score as the primary outcome measure. At a mean follow-up of 20 months (range 16–20 months), there was no difference between groups. Jo et al. [7] randomly assigned 48 patients with large to massive rotator cuff tears to PRP-augmented arthroscopic repair or conventional arthroscopic repair. They found that PRP application significantly improved retear rate (20.0 % vs. 55.6 %) and improved the cross-sectional area of the supraspinatus. In contrast, a cohort study by Bergeson et al. [8] found that patients who underwent arthroscopic rotator cuff repair with PRP matrix had a significantly higher retear rate (56 %) compared with controls (38 %). Moreover, postoperative functional scores were not significantly improved compared with controls. In a randomized controlled trial by Rodeo et al. [9] in which 40 patients received PRP-augmented repair and 39 patients received conventional repair, there were no differences in healing between groups, outcome scores, strength, and vascularity. Interestingly, PRP use was a significant predictor of tendon defect at 12 weeks. In another randomized control trial, Weber et al. [10] included 30 PRP patients and 30 controls and found no significant difference in ASES, VAS, and SST scores or recovery of motion. There were no differences in the rate of recurrent defect between groups assessed by MRI.

This inconclusive data underscores the need to clarify the optimal indication and use of PRP in rotator cuff repair through well-designed studies. Possible areas of investigation include identifying the optimal type of PRP, the timing and number of injections, and the effect of cytokines or other plasma proteins on PRP.

Patches

Mechanical augmentation of a rotator cuff repair is emerging as an important tool in the treatment of large or complex tears. Research has led to the development of natural and synthetic scaffolds derived from mammalian extracellular matrix (ECM), synthetic polymers, or a combination thereof. These materials are hypothesized to provide some degree of load sharing of forces across the tendon repair site, thus decreasing the likelihood of tendon retear [11]. It is also thought that the biomechanical advantage is only achieved if the devices have robust mechanical and suture-retention properties [12]. ECM-derived scaffolds are postulated to provide a conducive chemical and structural environment for repair healing and remodeling [13–15]. In contrast, synthetic scaffolds lack biological factors for repair healing, yet their mechanical strength may stabilize the repair construct until host tissue healing can occur [16].

Since ECM scaffolds are retrieved from different species and tissues, there is concern about the in vivo host response. In a rodent abdominal wall model, it was shown that all ECM scaffolds elicited an early, intense cellular response [17]. The removal of cells and cellular remnants from the ECM is thought to be crucial for a favorable host response. Overall, the host response is most likely dependent on the species of origin, tissue of origin, processing methods, methods of terminal sterilization, and mechanical loading environment [18].

For synthetic scaffolds, the sequence of host response commences with an acute inflammatory reaction, followed by chronic inflammation, and if the biomaterial is nondegradable granulation tissue and fibrous capsule formation [19, 20]. The duration and intensity of the host response are determined by its biomaterial composition and morphology. Unlike ECM scaffolds, there is little data on the host response to synthetic scaffolds used for rotator cuff repair. In a canine model, Derwin et al. [21] reported fibrous tissue ingrowth and an occasional presence of macrophages and foreign body giant cells. Cole et al. [22] found no evidence of inflammation at 6 weeks in a rat model. Currently, there are several synthetic scaffolds commercially available, and thus more studies are needed to fully assess the host response in the context of rotator cuff repair.

Large preclinical animal studies on ECM scaffolds (Restore, Zimmer Collagen Repair, GraftJacket) have reported generally good histologic outcomes, tendon-like remodeling, but little biomechanical improvement of the repair construct [23–26]. In contrast, synthetic scaffolds X-Repair and Biomerix RCR Patch have shown a biocompatible host response and significant improvement in the mechanical strength of the repair [21, 27].

While these preclinical studies are promising, clinical use of scaffolds in humans has raised concern in some instances [28–32]. The American Academy of Orthopedic Surgeons currently does not recommend the use of the non-cross-linked porcine small intestinal submucosa Restore™ for the treatment of rotator cuff tears in humans because of a severe, sterile postoperative inflammatory reaction documented in 20–30 % of patients [33, 34]. Better clinical outcomes, however, have been reported in other studies. Barber and colleagues [35] recently performed a prospective randomized controlled trial using GraftJacket for chronic two-tendon tears and reported significantly better ASES and constant scores and a significantly better healing rate compared to controls. Additionally, Hirooka et al. [36] and Audenaert et al. [37] both reported good clinical outcomes using synthetic scaffolds in large rotator cuff repairs at 44 and 43 months follow-up, respectively. In a recent study,

Encalada-Diaz et al. [16] used the Biomerix RCR Patch in 10 patients undergoing open repair of full-thickness tears of the supraspinatus or infraspinatus tendon. There was significant improvement in outcome scores at 1-year follow-up, although ultrasound and MRI demonstrated a 10 % failure rate.

Indications for the Use of Patches in the Treatment of Massive Rotator Cuff Repairs

In the setting of massive tears, patches are not indicated nor recommended for use as gapspanning devices. Patches should be used for augmentation only, particularly in the setting of large to massive tears that may be less likely to heal. We prefer to augment with patches in the setting of revision repairs and/or in those situations in which the patient's ability to heal may be compromised (i.e., diabetes).

Surgical Technique

Technique

Patients are positioned in the beach chair position. After the administration of regional anesthesia, the arm is prepped and draped sterilely. A standard posterior portal to the glenohumeral joint is established, and a thorough diagnostic arthroscopy is performed. Concomitant pathology is addressed, after which attention is turned to the rotator cuff. In the setting of massive tears, it is possible that extensive mobilization and even marginal convergence sutures are necessary. Once the torn tendons are mobilized enough to bring the edge back to the native footprint on the greater tuberosity, the repair construct is created.

When augmenting with a patch, a transosseous suture bridge technique is used for the repair. The first row of anchors is placed just lateral to the articular margin of the humeral head. Sutures from these medial anchors are placed in mattress fashion through the torn cuff. Arthroscopic knots are tied to secure the tendon to the medial aspect of the tuberosity. The

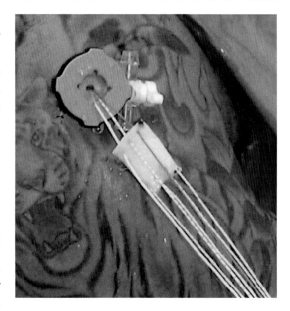

Fig. 6.1 View of the lateral aspect of the shoulder. Different-colored sutures from the medial row anchor/aspect of tendon through the patch

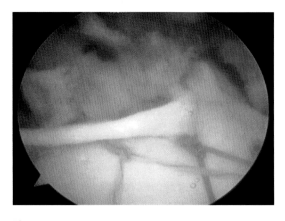

Fig. 6.2 Patch secured to medial aspect of tendon

strands of suture are not cut; instead they are brought out the lateral portal and sutured through what will be the medial aspect of the graft outside of the cannula (Fig. 6.1).

Once the medial sutures are passed through the graft outside the cannula, the graft is slid down the lateral cannula on top of the rotator cuff. It helps to use different colored sutures anteriorly and posteriorly so that the graft can be oriented appropriately in the subacromial space. Knots are tied to secure the graft to the tendon medially (Fig. 6.2).

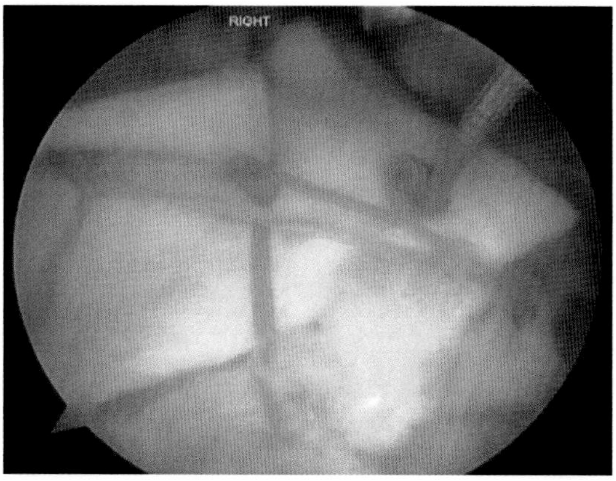

Fig. 6.3 Final construct with patch being incorporated over the tendon in a transosseous suture bridge repair construct

The sutures are then brought out laterally over the top of the patch/cuff and placed through a knotless anchor laterally (Fig. 6.3).

Postoperatively, patients are kept immobilized in an abduction sling for 4 weeks. This is followed by physical therapy for range of motion. At 3 months, strengthening is initiated.

Future Directions: Cytokines and Cells

Research has shown that growth factors and cytokines can be manipulated to enhance the healing process. PDGF-β has been found to promote fibroblast chemotaxis and proliferative activity, macrophage activation, extracellular matrix production, angiogenesis, and collagen synthesis [38]. It has also been demonstrated that PDGF-β enhances the proliferation of bone cells, which can improve the biochemical, mechanical, and structural properties of the healing site [39].

In addition to inducing osteoclast formation and bone resorption, TGF-β can enhance the proliferative activity of fibroblasts and stimulate the synthesis of type I collagen and fibronectin. TGF-β is not only found during normal fetal tendon development but also in the differentiation of scar tissue during tendon-to-bone healing. The type of healing that occurs depends on the ratio of different isoforms expressed, with TGF-β1 associated with scar-mediated healing and TGF-β3 associated with tissue regeneration and "scarless" healing [40]. When TGF-β1 is expressed during the inflammatory phase of tendon healing, there is stimulation of collagen synthesis, cell proliferation, and cell migration. Ultimately, this results in the formation of scar tissue. On the other hand, TGF-β3 expression has been linked to the development of the enthesis during prenatal stages as well as to the reduction in scar tissue formation after healing in adult wounds or tendon repairs [40, 41].

Bone morphogenetic proteins (BMP) are cytokines normally expressed during embryonic development, which participate in fibrocartilage tendon formation via a series of physiologically orchestrated signals. In particular, BMPs 2–7 have good osteoinductive properties. In contrast, recombinant human BMPs (rhBMP) 12, 13, and 14 have significantly different biologic activity that may have increased clinical benefit. These BMPs are expressed at the tendon interface during embryonic development and are primarily involved in the formation of fibrocartilage and tendon.

Lastly, FGF, expressed by fibroblasts and inflammatory cells, is involved in the promotion of cellular migration and angiogenesis to aid in proliferation and remodeling at the site of tendon repair [42].

Preclinical work on the use of growth factors to enhance tendon healing reveals a positive trend. Rodeo et al. [43] used a mixture of osteoinductive growth factors (BMP 2–7, FGF, TGF-β) in a sheep rotator cuff repair model. Biomechanical testing showed a stronger repair and increased bone and soft tissue formation at the repair site. Seeherman et al. [44] delivered rhBMP-12 via a type I/III collagen sponge to a sheep rotator cuff repair. Results showed a significantly greater load to failure and stiffness compared to controls. Histologic analysis demonstrated reestablishment of the collagen fiber continuity between the bone and fibrovascular interface scar tissue and increased glycosaminoglycan content in the rhBMP-12-treated specimens. In a rat model of rotator cuff repair augmented with FGF-2, Ide et al. [45] showed improved biomechanical and histologic outcomes at 2 weeks. However, there were no differences between experimental and control groups at 4 or 6 weeks. Uggen et al. [46] transduced rat tendon fibroblasts with PDGF and found increased DNA and collagen synthesis in transduced fibroblasts. Additionally, in a chronic rotator cuff repair model in rats, there was improved histology and biomechanics in the PDGF group. Hee et al. [47] used a sheep rotator cuff repair model with PDGF-BB + type I collagen matrix. They found an increase in ultimate load to failure in two middle dosages of PDGF. However, the highest dose group of PDGF had inferior results indicating a potential negative feedback loop and the need to elucidate an ideal concentration.

Stem Cell Therapy

Stem cells are undifferentiated, unspecialized cells that have the potential to be expanded and differentiated into various cell types in the body. When implanted, stem cells may function by direct participation in the repair process, a paracrine effect by stimulating other local (or distant) host cells, or an anti-inflammatory/immunomodulatory role. Stem cell-based approaches may be useful for augmentation of tendon-to-bone healing, tendon-to-tendon healing, and muscle regeneration and possibly reversal of fatty infiltration and muscle atrophy. Studies have indicated potential for stem cells to improve tendon healing. Ni et al. [48] created a rat patellar tendon window defect model and delivered tendon-derived stem cells in a fibrin glue carrier. The tendon-derived stem cells significantly enhanced tendon healing as evidenced by increased collagen fiber alignment and a significantly higher ultimate stress and Young's modulus. Nixon et al. [49] isolated stem cells from adipose tissue and induced tendonitis in eight horses. Forty-two days after injection of the stem cells, there was reduced inflammatory cell infiltrate and significant improvement in tendon fiber architecture and organization.

It is likely that stem cells alone may not be sufficient for healing. In a rat rotator cuff model in which animals received bone marrow-derived mesenchymal stem cells in a fibrin carrier, Gulotta et al. [50] showed that there was no difference in fibrocartilage formation, collagen fiber organization, and biomechanical strength of the repairs, peak stress to failure, or stiffness. They concluded that the repair site may lack the cellular and/or molecular signals necessary to induce appropriate differentiation of transplanted cells. In another study, this group modified mesenchymal stem cells with membrane type 1 matrix metalloproteinase, a gene upregulated during embryogenesis in areas that develop into tendon-bone insertion sites. At 4 weeks, the modified stem cells had significantly more fibrocartilage, higher ultimate load to failure, higher ultimate stress to failure, and higher stiffness values compared with the unmodified stem cells [51]. A subsequent study by Gulotta et al. transduced stem cells with scleraxis, a transcription factor that is thought to direct tendon development during embryogenesis. Results at 4 weeks were similar to the previous study, and the authors concluded mesenchymal stem cells genetically modified with scleraxis can augment rotator cuff healing at early time points [52].

Scaffolds may provide further enhancement of cell-based approaches. In a rabbit model, Yokoya et al. [53] reconstructed a surgically created defect in the infraspinatus tendon with a polyglycolic acid (PGA) sheet seeded with MSCs or PGA alone. Their findings showed that the MSC group had a more consistent restoration of fibrocartilage and Sharpey's fibers, improved type I to type III collagen ratio, and better tensile strength than PGA alone or control groups. However, the addition of PRP to patches does not appear to confer significant additive healing effect according to a recent study. In their rabbit model, Chung et al. [54] demonstrated that the local administration of PRP on repaired supraspinatus tendon enhanced biological tendon-to-bone healing and increased the load to failure of the repaired rotator cuff; however, porcine dermal collagen graft augmentation did not improve the biological and mechanical properties.

There is ample opportunity for impactful research in the cell-based treatment of rotator cuff tears. These approaches may be improved by targeted manipulation of the cells through culture conditions or sorting them by methods such as flow cytometry. Determining the optimal timing, concentration, and combination of different growth factors with stem cells would yield useful clinical information [55–57]. Another strategy to improve biologic augmentation involves gene therapy. For example, matrix metalloproteinase 3 has been identified as a candidate gene to enhance tendon healing through altering the postoperative/post-injury catabolic process. In sum, enhanced biological healing of the rotator cuff remains elusive, but future research should seek to find optimal methods for acquiring, processing, delivering, and maintaining autologous pluripotential cells within the healing zone [58].

Conclusion

As our understanding of the biology of healing improves, the hope is that we will be able to manipulate the rotator cuff repair milieu to improve outcomes following rotator cuff repair. In the future, this will likely come in the form of cellular strategies. At this point though, options to biologically enhance repair constructs are basically limited to platelet rich plasma and patches. To date, results of PRP augmentation in the setting of large rotator cuff repairs are not very promising. Patches can help when used in the appropriate setting.

Acknowledgement Figures courtesy of Gary Gartsman MD.

References

1. Nho SJ, Delos D, Yadav H, et al. Biomechanical and biologic augmentation for the treatment of massive rotator cuff tears. Am J Sports Med. 2010;38(3):619–29. doi:10.1177/0363546509343199.

2. American Academy of Orthopedic Surgeons. Research statistics on rotator cuff repairs, national inpatient sample, 1998–2004. The Agency for Healthcare Research and Quality. 2006.

3. Galatz LM, Ball CM, Teefey SA, Middleton WD, Yamaguchi K. The outcome and repair integrity of completely arthroscopically repaired large and massive rotator cuff tears. J Bone Joint Surg Am. 2004; 86-A(2):219–24.

4. Frank JB, ElAttrache NS, Dines JS, Blackburn A, Crues J, Tibone JE. Repair site integrity after arthroscopic transosseous-equivalent suture-bridge rotator cuff repair. Am J Sports Med. 2008;36(8):1496–503. doi:10.1177/0363546507313574.

5. Barber FA. Platelet-rich plasma for rotator cuff repair. Sports Med Arthrosc Rev. 2013;21(4):199–205. doi:10.1097/JSA.0b013e31828a7c6a.

6. Castricini R, Longo UG, De Benedetto M, et al. Platelet-rich plasma augmentation for arthroscopic rotator cuff repair: a randomized controlled trial. Am J Sports Med. 2011;39(2):258–65. doi:10.1177/0363546510390780.

7. Jo CH, Shin JS, Lee YG, et al. Platelet-rich plasma for arthroscopic repair of large to massive rotator cuff tears: a randomized, single-blind, parallel-group trial. Am J Sports Med. 2013;41(10):2240–8. doi:10.1177/0363546513497925.

8. Bergeson AG, Tashjian RZ, Greis PE, Crim J, Stoddard GJ, Burks RT. Effects of platelet-rich fibrin matrix on repair integrity of at-risk rotator cuff tears. Am J Sports Med. 2012;40(2):286–93. doi:10.1177/0363546511424402.

9. Rodeo SA, Delos D, Williams RJ, Adler RS, Pearle A, Warren RF. The effect of platelet-rich fibrin matrix on rotator cuff tendon healing: a prospective, randomized clinical study. Am J Sports Med. 2012;40(6):1234–41. doi:10.1177/0363546512442924.

10. Weber SC, Kauffman JI, Parise C, Weber SJ, Katz SD. Platelet-rich fibrin matrix in the management of arthroscopic repair of the rotator cuff: a prospective, randomized, double-blinded study. Am J Sports Med. 2013;41(2):263–70. doi:10.1177/0363546512467621.

11. Aurora A, McCarron JA, van den Bogert AJ, Gatica JE, Iannotti JP, Derwin KA. The biomechanical role of scaffolds in augmented rotator cuff tendon repairs. J Shoulder Elbow Surg. 2012;21(8):1064–71. doi:10.1016/j.jse.2011.05.014.

12. Derwin KA, Badylak SF, Steinmann SP, Iannotti JP. Extracellular matrix scaffold devices for rotator cuff repair. J Shoulder Elbow Surg. 2010;19(3):467–76. doi:10.1016/j.jse.2009.10.020.

13. Brown BN, Valentin JE, Stewart-Akers AM, McCabe GP, Badylak SF. Macrophage phenotype and remodeling outcomes in response to biologic scaffolds with and without a cellular component. Biomaterials. 2009;30(8):1482–91. doi:10.1016/j.biomaterials.2008.11.040.

14. Hodde JP, Ernst DMJ, Hiles MC. An investigation of the long-term bioactivity of endogenous growth factor in OASIS Wound Matrix. J Wound Care. 2005; 14(1):23–5.

15. Hodde JP, Record RD, Liang HA, Badylak SF. Vascular endothelial growth factor in porcine-derived extracellular matrix. Endothelium. 2001; 8(1):11–24.

16. Encalada-Diaz I, Cole BJ, Macgillivray JD, et al. Rotator cuff repair augmentation using a novel polycarbonate polyurethane patch: preliminary results at

12 months' follow-up. J Shoulder Elbow Surg. 2011;20(5):788–94. doi:10.1016/j.jse.2010.08.013.

17. Valentin JE, Badylak JS, McCabe GP, Badylak SF. Extracellular matrix bioscaffolds for orthopaedic applications. A comparative Histologic study. J Bone Joint Surg Am. 2006;88(12):2673–86. doi:10.2106/JBJS.E.01008.

18. Ricchetti ET, Aurora A, Iannotti JP, Derwin KA. Scaffold devices for rotator cuff repair. J Shoulder Elbow Surg. 2012;21(2):251–65. doi:10.1016/j.jse.2011.10.003.

19. Anderson JM, Rodriguez A, Chang DT. Foreign body reaction to biomaterials. Semin Immunol. 2008;20(2):86–100. doi:10.1016/j.smim.2007.11.004.

20. Mikos A, McIntire L, Anderson J, Babensee J. Host response to tissue engineered devices. Adv Drug Deliv Rev. 1998;33(1–2):111–39.

21. Derwin KA, Codsi MJ, Milks RA, Baker AR, McCarron JA, Iannotti JP. Rotator cuff repair augmentation in a canine model with use of a woven poly-L-lactide device. J Bone Joint Surg. 2009;91(5):1159–71. doi:10.2106/JBJS.H.00775.

22. Cole BJ, Gomoll AH, Yanke A, et al. Biocompatibility of a polymer patch for rotator cuff repair. Knee Surg Sports Traumatol Arthrosc. 2007;15(5):632–7. doi:10.1007/s00167-006-0187-6.

23. Adams JE, Zobitz ME, Reach JS, An K-N, Steinmann SP. Rotator cuff repair using an acellular dermal matrix graft: an in vivo study in a canine model. Arthroscopy. 2006;22(7):700–9. doi:10.1016/j.arthro.2006.03.016.

24. Dejardin LM, Arnoczky SP, Ewers BJ, Haut RC, Clarke RB. Tissue-engineered rotator cuff tendon using porcine small intestine submucosa. Histologic and mechanical evaluation in dogs. Am J Sports Med. 2001;29(2):175–84.

25. Nicholson GP, Breur GJ, Van Sickle D, Yao JQ, Kim J, Blanchard CR. Evaluation of a cross-linked acellular porcine dermal patch for rotator cuff repair augmentation in an ovine model. J Shoulder Elbow Surg. 2007;16(5 Suppl):S184–90. doi:10.1016/j.jse.2007.03.010.

26. Schlegel TF, Hawkins RJ, Lewis CW, Motta T, Turner AS. The effects of augmentation with Swine small intestine submucosa on tendon healing under tension: histologic and mechanical evaluations in sheep. Am J Sports Med. 2006;34(2):275–80. doi:10.1177/0363546505279912.

27. Schepull T, Kvist J, Andersson C, Aspenberg P. Mechanical properties during healing of Achilles tendon ruptures to predict final outcome: a pilot Roentgen stereophotogrammetric analysis in 10 patients. BMC Musculoskelet Disord. 2007;8(1):116. doi:10.1186/1471-2474-8-116.

28. Badhe SP, Lawrence TM, Smith FD, Lunn PG. An assessment of porcine dermal xenograft as an augmentation graft in the treatment of extensive rotator cuff tears. J Shoulder Elbow Surg. 2008;17 (1 Suppl):35S–9. doi:10.1016/j.jse.2007.08.005.

29. Halder A, Zobitz ME, Schultz E, An KN. Structural properties of the subscapularis tendon. J Orthop Res. 2000;18(5):829–34. doi:10.1002/jor.1100180522.

30. Metcalf MH, Savoie FH, Kellum B. Surgical technique for xenograft (SIS) augmentation of rotator-cuff repairs. Oper Tech Orthop. 2002;12(3):204–8.

31. Sclamberg SG, Tibone JE, Itamura JM, Kasraeian S. Six-month magnetic resonance imaging follow-up of large and massive rotator cuff repairs reinforced with porcine small intestinal submucosa. J Shoulder Elbow Surg. 2004;13(5):538–41. doi:10.1016/S1058274604001193.

32. Soler JA, Gidwani S, Curtis MJ. Early complications from the use of porcine dermal collagen implants (Permacol) as bridging constructs in the repair of massive rotator cuff tears. A report of 4 cases. Acta Orthop Belg. 2007;73(4):432–6.

33. Iannotti JP, Codsi MJ, Kwon YW, Derwin K, Ciccone J, Brems JJ. Porcine small intestine submucosa augmentation of surgical repair of chronic two-tendon rotator cuff tears. A randomized, controlled trial. J Bone Joint Surg Am. 2006;88(6):1238–44.

34. Walton JR, Bowman NK, Khatib Y, Linklater J, Murrell GAC. Restore orthobiologic implant: not recommended for augmentation of rotator cuff repairs. J Bone Joint Surg Am. 2007;89(4):786–91. doi:10.2106/JBJS.F.00315.

35. Barber FA, Burns JP, Deutsch A, Labbé MR, Litchfield RB. A prospective, randomized evaluation of acellular human dermal matrix augmentation for arthroscopic rotator cuff repair. Arthroscopy. 2012;28(1):8–15. doi:10.1016/j.arthro.2011.06.038.

36. Hirooka A, Yoneda M, Wakaitani S, et al. Augmentation with a Gore-Tex patch for repair of large rotator cuff tears that cannot be sutured. J Orthop Sci. 2002;7(4):451–6. doi:10.1007/s007760200078.

37. Audenaert E, Van Nuffel J, Schepens A, Verhelst M, Verdonk R. Reconstruction of massive rotator cuff lesions with a synthetic interposition graft: a prospective study of 41 patients. Knee Surg Sports Traumatol Arthrosc. 2006;14(4):360–4. doi:10.1007/s00167-005-0689-7.

38. Gulotta LV, Rodeo SA. Growth factors for rotator cuff repair. Clin Sports Med. 2009;28(1):13–23. doi:10.1016/j.csm.2008.09.002.

39. Chan BP, Fu SC, Qin L, Rolf C, Chan KM. Supplementation-time dependence of growth factors in promoting tendon healing. Clin Orthop Relat Res. 2006;448:240–7. doi:10.1097/01.blo.0000205875.97468.e4.

40. Kovacevic D, Fox AJ, Bedi A, et al. Calcium-phosphate matrix with or without TGF-β3 improves tendon-bone healing after rotator cuff repair. Am J Sports Med. 2011;39(4):811–9. doi:10.1177/0363546511399378.

41. Galatz L, Rothermich S, VanderPloeg K, Petersen B, Sandell L, Thomopoulos S. Development of the supraspinatus tendon-to-bone insertion: localized expression of extracellular matrix and growth factor genes. J Orthop Res. 2007;25(12):1621–8. doi:10.1002/jor.20441.

42. Carpenter JE, Thomopoulos S, Flanagan CL, DeBano CM, Soslowsky LJ. Rotator cuff defect healing: a biomechanical and histologic analysis in an animal model. J Shoulder Elbow Surg. 1998;7(6):599–605.

43. Rodeo SA, Potter HG, Kawamura S, Turner AS, Kim HJ, Atkinson BL. Biologic augmentation of rotator cuff tendon-healing with use of a mixture of osteoinductive growth factors. J Bone Joint Surg. 2007;89(11):2485–97. doi:10.2106/JBJS.C.01627.

44. Seeherman HJ, Archambault JM, Rodeo SA, et al. rhBMP-12 accelerates healing of rotator cuff repairs in a sheep model. J Bone Joint Surg. 2008;90(10): 2206–19.

45. Ide J, Kikukawa K, Hirose J, Iyama K-I, Sakamoto H, Mizuta H. The effects of fibroblast growth factor-2 on rotator cuff reconstruction with acellular dermal matrix grafts. Arthroscopy. 2009;25(6):608–16. doi:10.1016/j.arthro.2008.11.011.

46. Uggen JC, Dines J, Uggen CW, et al. Tendon gene therapy modulates the local repair environment in the shoulder. J Am Osteopath Assoc. 2005;105(1):20–1.

47. Hee CK, Dines JS, Dines DM, et al. Augmentation of a rotator cuff suture repair using rhPDGF-BB and a type I bovine collagen matrix in an ovine model. Am J Sports Med. 2011;39(8):1630–9. doi:10.1177/ 0363546511404942.

48. Ni M, Lui PPY, Rui YF, et al. Tendon-derived stem cells (TDSCs) promote tendon repair in a rat patellar tendon window defect model. J Orthop Res. 2012;30(4):613–9. doi:10.1002/jor.21559.

49. Nixon AJ, Dahlgren LA, Haupt JL, Yeager AE, Ward DL. Effect of adipose-derived nucleated cell fractions on tendon repair in horses with collagenase-induced tendinitis. Am J Vet Res. 2008;69(7):928–37. doi:10.2460/ajvr.69.7.928.

50. Gulotta LV, Kovacevic D, Ehteshami JR, Dagher E, Packer JD, Rodeo SA. Application of bone marrow-derived mesenchymal stem cells in a rotator cuff repair model. Am J Sports Med. 2009;37(11):2126–33. doi:10.1177/0363546509339582.

51. Gulotta LV, Kovacevic D, Montgomery S, Ehteshami JR, Packer JD, Rodeo SA. Stem cells genetically modified with the developmental gene MT1-MMP improve regeneration of the supraspinatus tendon-to-bone insertion site. Am J Sports Med. 2010;38(7):1429–37. doi:10.1177/0363546510361235.

52. Gulotta LV, Kovacevic D, Packer JD, Deng XH, Rodeo SA. Bone marrow-derived mesenchymal stem cells transduced with scleraxis improve rotator cuff healing in a rat model. Am J Sports Med. 2011;39(6):1282–9. doi:10.1177/0363546510395485.

53. Yokoya S, Mochizuki Y, Natsu K, Omae H, Nagata Y, Ochi M. Rotator cuff regeneration using a bioabsorbable material with bone marrow-derived mesenchymal stem cells in a rabbit model. Am J Sports Med. 2012;40(6):1259–68. doi:10.1177/0363546512442343.

54. Chung SW, Song BW, Kim YH, Park KU, Oh JH. Effect of platelet-rich plasma and porcine dermal collagen graft augmentation for rotator cuff healing in a rabbit model. Am J Sports Med. 2013;41(12): 2909–18. doi:10.1177/0363546513503810.

55. Butler DL, Juncosa-Melvin N, Boivin GP, et al. Functional tissue engineering for tendon repair: a multidisciplinary strategy using mesenchymal stem cells, bioscaffolds, and mechanical stimulation. J Orthop Res. 2008;26(1):1–9. doi:10.1002/jor.20456.

56. Shea KP, McCarthy MB, Ledgard F, Arciero C, Chowaniec D, Mazzocca AD. Human tendon cell response to 7 commercially available extracellular matrix materials: an in vitro study. Arthroscopy. 2010;26(9):1181–8. doi:10.1016/j.arthro.2010.01.020.

57. Derwin KA, Baker AR, Spragg RK, Leigh DR, Iannotti JP. Commercial extracellular matrix scaffolds for rotator cuff tendon repair. Biomechanical, biochemical, and cellular properties. J Bone Joint Surg Am. 2006;88(12):2665–72.

58. Arce G, Bak K, Bain G, et al. Management of disorders of the rotator cuff: proceedings of the ISAKOS upper extremity committee consensus meeting. 2013;29: 1840–50. doi:10.1016/j.arthro.2013.07.265. Elsevier.

Latissimus Dorsi Tendon Transfer

Moira M. McCarthy and Russell F. Warren

Pearls and Pitfalls

Pearls

- Proper patient selection is of utmost importance. Ideal candidate will be men with posterosuperior rotator cuff tears, an intact subscapularis, and retain the ability to elevate to horizontal.
- Understanding the anatomy and location of the thoracodorsal, radial, and axillary nerve is important to avoid injury.
- Maximal shoulder internal rotation will aid in dissecting the latissimus dorsi off its humeral insertion and will protect the radial nerve.

Pitfalls

- Managing Patient Expectations. This tendon transfer is not perfect but can provide pain relief and improved function when performed in the appropriately selected patient with reasonable postoperative goals and expectations.
- Maximal internal rotation with tenotomy is important to ensure enough tendon length for attachment on the footprint of the greater tuberosity.
- Although lengthening of the transferred tendon with allograft augmentation is an option, we do not recommend it.

Background

Massive, irreparable rotator cuff tears represent a small percentage of all rotator cuff tears, but represent a difficult clinical problem. Of all rotator cuff tears, approximately 95 % are amenable to surgical repair [1]. Just because a cuff tear is massive, however, does not mean it is necessarily irreparable. Some massive cuff tears can be repaired with good results [2]. However, massive cuff tears when associated with poor quality tissue, significant muscle atrophy, and the inability to adequately mobilize cuff tissue are considered

M.M. McCarthy, MD (✉)
Sports Medicine and Shoulder Surgery, Hospital for Special Surgery, 535 E 70th Street, New York, NY 10021, USA
e-mail: mccarthymo@hss.edu

R.F. Warren, MD
Department of Orthopaedics, Hospital for Special Surgery, 535 E 70th Street, New York, NY 10021, USA
e-mail: warrenr@hss.edu

irreparable and require an alternative treatment method [3, 4]. One definition of a massive, irreparable rotator cuff tear is a tear that involves at least two tendons that cannot be repaired with the arm in less than 60° of abduction [5]. Others have defined massive rotator cuff tears as those with a tear diameter of greater than 5 cm [6].

Posterosuperior rotator cuff tears, involving the supraspinatus, infraspinatus, and, less commonly, the teres minor, are the most common configuration of massive, irreparable rotator cuff tears and lead to loss of active external rotation and the inability to position and stabilize the arm in space. Patients with massive rotator cuff tears can have stable glenohumeral abduction without excessive superior translation if the remaining intact cuff generates force sufficient to counteract the deltoid [7]. With a 6 or 7 cm tear, the increased force requirements are 50 %, but with an 8 cm tear, the increased force requirements are 80 % [7]. Some patients may be amenable to conservative treatment initially, but ultimately some will decompensate when either the tear size increases due to the increased force or the remaining cuff becomes deconditioned. This can lead to significant functional impairment with daily activities as well as chronic, disabling pain that may not respond to conservative management [8].

The most common tendon transfer for rotator cuff deficiency, in isolation or in combination with other tendon transfers, is the latissimus dorsi tendon transfer. Gerber et al. [5] described the latissimus dorsi tendon transfer for the treatment of irreparable, posterosuperior rotator cuff tears in 1988 and reported pain relief and functional improvements without any significant complications. This tendon transfer for irreparable rotator cuff tears was adapted from the treatment of Erb's brachial plexus palsy and is designed to provide containment of the humeral head with the added benefit of providing an external rotation force. The containment of the humeral head increases the efficiency of the remaining rotator cuff musculature and the deltoid and allows improved glenohumeral motion especially with regard to anterior elevation [5, 9, 10]. The results from this procedure have been mixed, and many studies have been conducted

looking at the anatomy of the transfer and the technical difficulties associated with the surgical procedure and its modifications [11–16].

Indications and Contraindications

Indications and contraindications for latissimus dorsi tendon transfer have been well reported based on clinical observations and studies [5, 10, 17]. Tables 7.1 and 7.2 list indications and contraindications, respectively. This tendon transfer is indicated in patients with pain refractory to conservative management, significant weakness, and dysfunction of the shoulder in the setting of a massive, posterosuperior rotator cuff tear with minimal or no arthritis. Although there are no strict age or gender criteria, younger male patients are preferred for this technique because they have better outcomes postoperatively. Pain alone in the setting of a massive rotator cuff tear is not necessarily an indication for a latissimus dorsi tendon transfer. An attempt must be made to treat each patient with an appropriate course of physical

Table 7.1 Surgical indications for latissimus dorsi tendon transfer

Refractory pain
Significant dysfunction and disability
Posterosuperior, massive rotator cuff tear or failed prior repair that is no longer amenable to repair or has a high likelihood of failure with repair
Minimal radiographic evidence of osteoarthritis or anteroposterior instability
Fatty degeneration > stage 2 of supraspinatus and/or infraspinatus muscles

Table 7.2 Contraindications to latissimus dorsi tendon transfer

Anterosuperior rotator cuff tears
Subscapularis insufficiency
Static or dynamic anterior or posterior instability
Advanced osteoarthritis
Inflammatory arthritis
Axillary nerve injury
Deltoid insufficiency
Comorbid conditions negatively impacting postoperative rehabilitation potential

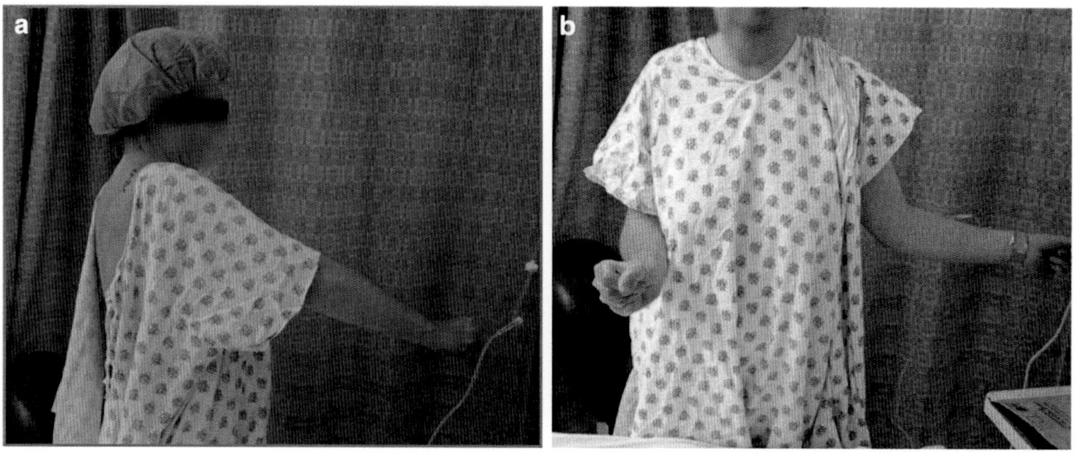

Fig. 7.1 Clinical photo of a patient with a massive rotator cuff tear and minimal (**a**) forward elevation and (**b**) external rotation (Figure taken with permission from Pearle et al. [18])

therapy, anti-inflammatory pain medications as tolerated, and injections to determine what role the pain is playing in the dysfunction of the shoulder.

Function and range of motion of the shoulder are essential to daily activities and often represent significant disability when absent. The degree of weakness and dysfunction is essential in the decision-making process (Fig. 7.1). With a massive posterosuperior tear, there will be a lag between passive and active external rotation. Evaluation of forward elevation is an essential component to determine shoulder function. With mild to moderate weakness, a latissimus dorsi tendon transfer is expected to provide sufficient power to elevate the arm against gravity above shoulder level. With severe weakness or pseudoparalysis, a latissimus dorsi tendon transfer is less predictable. In most patients with pseudoparalysis, it will not reliably provide effective overhead motion.

In addition to a careful and thorough physical examination, radiographic evaluation is essential. Standard radiographs including a true anteroposterior with the arm in neutral rotation are essential. Radiographs should be evaluated for the presence of osteophytes and joint space narrowing. The axillary radiograph should be evaluated to assess whether there are any anteroposterior instability, posterior subluxation, and evidence of arthritis. Superior humeral head migration, as seen with massive rotator cuff tears and cuff arthropathy, reduces the efficiency of the deltoid as a shoulder abductor and increases impingement. Superior humeral migration with an acromiohumeral distance of less than 5 cm is also a relative contraindication to a latissimus dorsi tendon transfer. Advanced osteoarthritis and any inflammatory arthritic conditions are contraindications to latissimus dorsi tendon transfers. These patients are often better served with a joint arthroplasty such as a reverse total shoulder. An overall guideline is that patients aged 60 or older are probably better suited to a reverse total shoulder arthroplasty, whereas patients aged 40 to early 50s may be a candidate for latissimus transfer, pending the results of other studies. Advanced imaging such as MRI is necessary to assess the whether the rotator cuff can be primarily repaired. This is most reliably determined by evaluating muscle fatty infiltration within the muscle as described by Goutallier [19].

Strict contraindications include static or dynamic anteroposterior instability. Many studies, as discussed in the outcomes section, have been performed looking at the outcomes of patients with and without subscapularis function after latissimus dorsi tendon transfers. Subscapularis insufficiency leads to lower postoperative outcomes and is considered a contraindication to latissimus

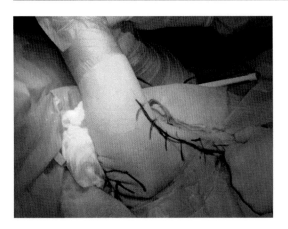

Fig. 7.2 Patient in the lateral decubitus position with the arm in abduction in an extremity holder. The extremity holder allows for easy manipulation of the arm, with specific respect to internal and external rotation (Figure taken with permission from Pearle et al. [18])

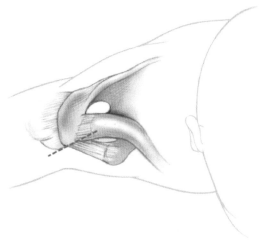

Fig. 7.3 The anterior incision is vertical and begins at the anterolateral edge of the acromion. The anterior deltoid raphe is split up to 5 cm distal to the acromion. The axillary nerve crosses more than 5 cm distal to the acromion (Figure taken with permission from Pearle et al. [18])

transfers. After a thorough discussion of patient history, activity level, and expectations of surgical outcome, decision to proceed with a latissimus dorsi tendon transfer should be made based on indications, pain, and disability refractory to conservative treatment.

Technique

The surgical procedure is a modification of the original description of the latissimus dorsi tendon transfer by Gerber et al. [5] and has been previously reported by Pearle et al. [14, 18]. Regional anesthesia is performed prior to patient positioning. The patient is positioned in the lateral decubitus with sufficient access to the entire scapula and latissimus dorsi muscle belly. The entire limb and hemithorax are prepped and draped. A complete examination under anesthesia is performed with special focus on the stability of the joint as well as passive range of motion. The arm is positioned using the Spider limb positioner (Smith and Nephew, Andover, MA) which allows maintenance of limb position throughout the procedure (Fig. 7.2). The bony landmarks of the shoulder including the anterior and posterior acromion, acromioclavicular joint, coracoid process, and clavicle are palpated and appropriately marked.

A two-incision technique is then performed. The rotator cuff is approached (Fig. 7.3) through a standard vertical incision starting at the anterolateral edge of the acromion. The anterior raphe of the deltoid is identified and divided up to 5 cm distal to the acromion where care is taken to avoid injuring the anterior branch of the axillary nerve. The anterior aspect of the deltoid is detached sharply from the acromion and an acromioplasty is performed when needed. A complete inspection of the rotator cuff tissue is performed with every effort made to mobilize all retracted cuff tissue, lyse adhesions, resect the coracohumeral ligament, release the capsule, and attempt any possible tension-free repairs. Care is taken to preserve the coracoacromial ligament. Upon confirmation that no appropriate repair can be performed, attention is turned toward the latissimus dorsi tendon transfer. Of note, a combination latissimus dorsi and teres major transfer can be performed. When both tendons are transferred, there is usually insufficient excursion to reach the superior aspect of the greater tuberosity. Instead, the tendons can be reattached to the posterolateral aspect of the proximal humeral, around the teres minor insertion site. Therefore, this technique is typically reserved for patients in which

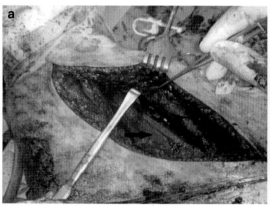

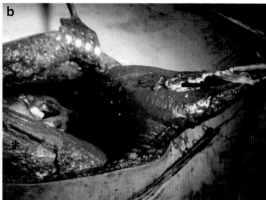

Fig. 7.4 Intraoperative photo of a patient in the lateral decubitus position with the arm in an extremity holder. (**a**) A 15 cm posterior incision is made along the border of the latissimus dorsi and is continued superiorly at the posterior axillary border. The muscle belly is dissected in a proximal direction. The interval between the teres major (*arrowhead*) and latissimus dorsi (*arrow*) is identified. (**b**) After the latissimus dorsi tendon (*arrow*) has been released. The thoracodorsal nerve and vessels (*arrowhead*) are identified. The teres major tendon (*asterisk*) remains attached in this specimen (Figure taken with permission from Pearle et al. [18])

external rotation weakness is their predominate complaint, and forward flexion remains fairly strong (which is a rare combination). The technique outlined here will discuss only isolated latissimus dorsi tendon transfers.

A posterior incision is used to harvest the latissimus dorsi tendon. A 15 cm incision over the lateral border of the latissimus dorsi and extending superiorly to the posterior border of the axilla is made (Fig. 7.4a). The latissimus dorsi muscle belly is identified posteroinferiorly and dissected in a proximal direction. The thoracodorsal nerve and vessels run on the undersurface of the latissimus dorsi muscle belly and must be protected throughout (Fig. 7.4b) to prevent postoperative denervation of the transferred muscle.

The next component of the procedure is critical to allow appropriate tendon transfer length as well as to avoid the neurovascular structures that are at risk with this procedure. The tendon of the latissimus dorsi muscle is found and traced laterally toward the humerus. As dissection is carried laterally, the tendon of the teres major is identified and the two tendons can be followed to their insertions on the anteromedial portion of the humerus (Fig. 7.5). The teres major has a very short tendon, and its insertion remains muscular until just before its insertion into the humeral. In comparison, the latissimus dorsi tendon is long

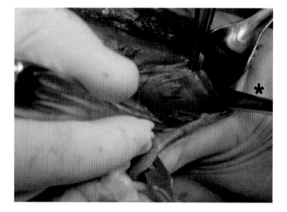

Fig. 7.5 Intraoperative photo of the right arm with the posterior incision exposed. The tendons of the teres major and latissimus dorsi (*arrow*) are identified and followed to their insertions on the anteromedial aspect of the humerus (*arrowhead*). The arm must be maximally internally rotated in the extremity holder to allow for a safe tenotomy directly from the humeral insertion (Figure taken with permission from Pearle et al. [18])

and flat and may be adherent to the undersurface of the teres major muscle. The latissimus dorsi is the most anterior tendon in the posterior axillary fold. During dissection of the tendinous insertions, it is imperative to maximally internally rotate the arm in the limb positioner to allow for a safe tenotomy that maximizes tendon length and places the radial nerve at less risk.

The anatomy of the latissimus dorsi and teres major tendons at their insertions has been well studied. In adults, the latissimus average width at insertion is 3.1 cm (2.4–4.8), average length is 8.4 cm (6.3–10.1), and the average distance from the humeral insertion to the thoracodorsal nerve is 13.1 cm (11.0–15.3) [14]. The latissimus and teres major tendons may either insert as separate tendons or may join and insert as a conjoint tendon which requires sharp dissection to separate [14]. Other important neurovascular structures including the radial nerve and axillary nerve must be appreciated during dissection. The radial nerve passes over the anterior surface of the tendons and, with the arm in neutral rotation and adduction, is 2.9 cm (2.0–4.0) medial to the humerus at the superior border of the latissimus tendon [14]. The axillary nerve is 1.4 cm (0.8–2.0) proximal to the superior edge of the teres major [14].

With the arm in maximal internal rotation, the latissimus tendon insertion can be sharply tenotomized safely from the humerus under direct visualization. Maximal internal rotation provides an additional 1.9 cm (1.5–2.4) of tendon tissue as compared to neutral rotation [18]. The posterior approach to the tendons for harvest provides visualization of a band of variable thickness just anterior to the tendon insertion. This band is the proximal aspect of the intermuscular septum and, when encountered, provides an additional landmark to ensure radial nerve protection.

The latissimus dorsi tendon and muscle are then mobilized from the chest wall (Fig. 7.6). The tendon is tagged with nonabsorbable sutures which provide traction to safely dissect the muscle from the chest wall. This axial dissection is performed until there is enough tendon excursion to reach the posterolateral border of the acromion. The average free musculotendinous length after mobilization is approximately 20 cm [18]. Of course, it is imperative during immobilization to ensure the safety and continuity of the neurovascular pedicle to the latissimus dorsi muscle to ensure appropriate function postoperatively.

The next step of the procedure is to pass the tendon under the deltoid to the position of attachment on the greater tuberosity. This "tunnel" for passage is created by identifying the

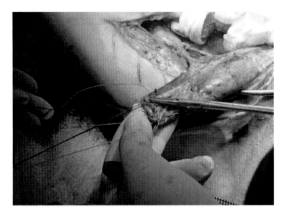

Fig. 7.6 Intraoperative photo of the right arm with the posterior incision exposed. The latissimus dorsi tendon was sutured in a Krakow pattern and mobilized for transfer (Figure taken with permission from Pearle et al. [18])

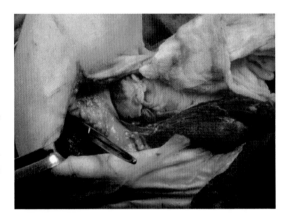

Fig. 7.7 Intraoperative photo of the right arm with the posterior incision exposed. The clamp is passed from the anterior to the posterior incision to grasp the sutures attached to the latissimus dorsi tendon. Care must be taken to avoid the axillary nerve and the quadrilateral space with passage of the clamp (Figure taken with permission from Pearle et al. [18])

plane between the posterior rotator cuff musculature and the posterior deltoid. With the posterior deltoid retracted laterally, a large, curved clamp is passed through the anterior incision, under the deltoid, and out the posterior incision. This provides a passage for the latissimus dorsi tendon (Fig. 7.7). The axillary nerve and its branches are at risk during this aspect of the procedure and must be avoided as the nerve exits the quadrilateral space and travels deep to the deltoid.

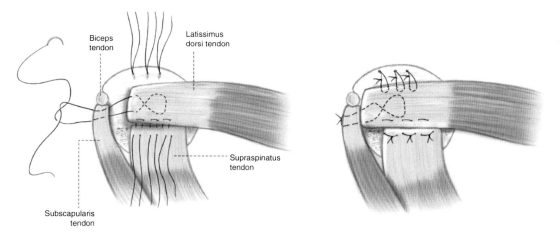

Fig. 7.8 The supraspinatus and infraspinatus are repaired to the transferred tendon if possible medially. The transferred latissimus dorsi tendon is sutured anteriorly to the superior border of the subscapularis muscle. Laterally, the transferred latissimus dorsi tendon is attached to the rotator cuff footprint with suture anchors (Figure taken with permission from Pearle et al. [18])

The plane between the deltoid and the posterior cuff, therefore, must be carefully and reliably identified because superficial deviation will place the axillary nerve and the superior lateral brachial cutaneous nerve at risk. The tendon is then passed by placing the previously placed tagging sutures in the clamp and withdrawing the clamp through the anterior incision. Suture anchors are used to secure the transferred latissimus dorsi tendon to the footprint attachment of the torn rotator cuff tendons (Fig. 7.8). The remainder of the previously mobilized rotator cuff tissue is used to augment the transfer and the anterior edge of the transferred tendon is sutured to the subscapularis tendon.

The patient is placed in an abduction sling with gentle pendulum exercises for 6 weeks. Passive and active-assist supine forward elevation are begun after 6 weeks. Therapists and surgeons must be careful to ensure that compensatory scapulothoracic shrugging does not occur when motion is initiated. Active supine range of motion followed by active motion and strengthening is performed beginning 12 weeks postoperatively. Close monitoring with a qualified therapist is essential to avoid postoperative complications.

Outcomes

The latissimus dorsi tendon transfer has been generally used as a salvage, non-arthroplasty treatment for massive, irreparable rotator cuff tears in shoulders without evidence of significant arthritis and in younger patients. The results of the studies on latissimus dorsi tendon transfers, in isolation or in combination with other tendon transfers, vary depending on a variety of different patient variables.

In the original article describing the technique and outcomes, Gerber reported that patients gained an average of 50° of active elevation and 13° of active external rotation [5]. Importantly, he noted that a deficient subscapularis tendon was associated with poor outcomes [5]. Gerber's subsequent studies on the mid- and long-term follow-up of latissimus dorsi tendon transfer outcomes have shown significant improvements in pain relief, flexion, external rotation, and strength in abduction, but again poor outcomes when associated with subscapularis deficiency [8, 10].

The role of the subscapularis in the setting of a latissimus dorsi tendon transfer for a massive rotator cuff tear has been well reported in the literature. Biomechanically, the subscapularis provides the restraint to anterior translation and dislocation of the joint in the neutral and in the abducted and externally rotated arm [20]. When the latissimus tendon is transferred to a shoulder with a deficient subscapularis, the centering action of the humeral head with abduction and elevation does not occur and has been explained as a biomechanical analysis of the poor outcomes of the tendon transfer with subscapularis deficiency [20]. A recent systematic review [21] reported on nine studies [8, 10, 16, 22–27] evaluating outcomes in subscapularis-deficient patients with a latissimus transfer and all 59 patients had poor results. Gerber et al. [10] reported that the functional value of the shoulder with a latissimus transfer and a functional subscapularis was 82 %, whereas without a functional subscapularis it was only 48 %. Many authors agree that without a functional subscapularis, the latissimus tendon transfer is of no value and should not be used [10, 22]. Miniaci et al. [17], however, report good results in patients with a latissimus transfer even in the setting on a subscapularis tear and do not consider that a contraindication to tendon transfer.

Costouros et al. [28] reported that fatty infiltration of the teres minor tendon greater than stage 2 resulted in lower Constant scores with or without the presence of a tear of the teres minor tendon. All authors do not agree as Miniaci et al. [17] reported that the teres minor integrity was not necessary for good results.

Other prognostic factors associated with good outcomes for the latissimus dorsi tendon transfer include good preoperative active shoulder forward flexion and active external rotation as well as good strength [24]. Synchronous inphase contraction of the transferred latissimus dorsi tendon, although a variable finding, is associated with a better clinical result [24]. Lastly, female patients with poor preoperative shoulder function and muscle weakness have a greater risk for a poor clinical outcome [24].

The preoperative presence of osteoarthritis and the progression of arthritis are important outcome measures to assess for the latissimus dorsi tendon transfer. Gerber et al. [10] reported no progression of osteoarthritis in 14/16 shoulders and progression from mild to moderate in the other two shoulders. The degree of superior migration was related to the overall functional outcome in this study. Compared to normal shoulder outcome scores, shoulders with latissimus transfers without superior migration scored 90 %, with mild superior migration scored 77 %, and with severe superior migration scored 62 % [10]. Aoki et al. report similar outcomes of progression of arthritis with 7/12 showing no arthritis, 3 showing mild to severe progression, and 2 showing mild to moderate progression [22]. Several other authors reported that the degree of osteoarthritis increased and the mean acromiohumeral head distance decreased at follow-up [28–30]. Outcomes in patients with severe osteoarthritis and a latissimus transfer are worse than those with mild or moderate arthritis, but the differences are not statistically significant [29].

Warner et al. [26] compared the outcomes for patients who underwent a latissimus dorsi tendon transfer as a salvage procedure with those who underwent a primary reconstruction for an irreparable defect. Poor tendon quality, fatty degeneration of the muscle, and detachment of the deltoid insertion negatively affected the outcome. The tendon transfer ruptured in 44 % of the salvage group and only 17 % of the primary group. The average Constant scores were significantly better for the primary reconstruction group ($P < 0.05$) at 70 % versus 55 % for the salvage group. Irlenbusch et al. [25] reported similar results with lower outcome scores present in the revision setting compared to the primary setting. Debeer et al. [29], however, found no significant differences in outcomes between primary or revision surgery. They suggested that most of the prior repairs were done arthroscopically in their series and the preservation of deltoid integrity in the primary surgery was the factor that did not cause a significant difference in outcomes between primary and revision surgeries. Miniaci et al. [17] and Birmingham et al. [31] both reported good outcomes in the setting of salvage operations.

Conclusion

Irreparable rotator cuff tears that present with chronic debilitating pain, dysfunction, and weakness may be treated with a latissimus dorsi tendon transfer. With the appropriately selected patient, pain relief and improvements in forward flexion and external rotation can be expected after completion of long-term rehabilitation. The outcomes of the surgical procedure require knowledge and respect of the anatomy to preserve all neurovascular structures and appropriate patient selection for the latissimus dorsi tendon transfer. Subscapularis insufficiency, deltoid insufficiency, and severe osteoarthritis lead to worse outcomes with latissimus dorsi tendon transfers for massive rotator cuff tears, and patients with such conditions may be better served with a different surgical procedure.

References

1. Warner J, Gerber C. Treatment of massive rotator cuff tears: posterior-superior and anterior-superior. In: Iannotti J, editor. The rotator cuff: current concepts and complex problems. Rosemont: American Academy of Orthopaedic Surgeons; 1998. p. 59–94.
2. Cordasco FA, Bigliani LU. The rotator cuff. Large and massive tears. Technique of open repair. Orthop Clin North Am. 1997;28(2):179–93.
3. Neviaser JS, Neviaser RJ, Neviaser TJ. The repair of chronic massive ruptures of the rotator cuff of the shoulder by use of a freeze-dried rotator cuff. J Bone Joint Surg Am. 1978;60(5):681–4.
4. Rockwood Jr CA, Williams Jr GR, Burkhead Jr WZ. Debridement of degenerative, irreparable lesions of the rotator cuff. J Bone Joint Surg Am. 1995;77(6):857–66.
5. Gerber C, Vinh TS, Hertel R, et al. Latissimus dorsi transfer for the treatment of massive tears of the rotator cuff. A preliminary report. Clin Orthop Relat Res. 1988;(232):51–61.
6. DeOrio JK, Cofield RH. Results of a second attempt at surgical repair of a failed initial rotator-cuff repair. J Bone Joint Surg Am. 1984;66(4):563–7.
7. Hansen ML, Otis JC, Johnson JS, et al. Biomechanics of massive rotator cuff tears: implications for treatment. J Bone Joint Surg Am. 2008;90(2):316–25.
8. Gerber C, Maquieira G, Espinosa N. Latissimus dorsi transfer for the treatment of irreparable rotator cuff tears. J Bone Joint Surg Am. 2006;88(1):113–20.
9. Burkhart SS. Biomechanics of rotator cuff repair: converting the ritual to a science. Instr Course Lect. 1998;47:43–50.
10. Gerber C. Latissimus dorsi transfer for the treatment of irreparable tears of the rotator cuff. Clin Orthop Relat Res. 1992;(275):152–60.
11. Codsi MJ, Hennigan S, Herzog R, et al. Latissimus dorsi tendon transfer for irreparable posterosuperior rotator cuff tears. Surgical technique. J Bone Joint Surg Am. 2007;89(Suppl 2 Pt 1):1–9.
12. Lehmann LJ, Mauerman E, Strube T, et al. Modified minimally invasive latissimus dorsi transfer in the treatment of massive rotator cuff tears: a two-year follow-up of 26 consecutive patients. Int Orthop. 2010;34(3):377–83.
13. Morelli M, Nagamori J, Gilbart M, et al. Latissimus dorsi tendon transfer for massive irreparable cuff tears: an anatomic study. J Shoulder Elbow Surg. 2008;17(1):139–43.
14. Pearle AD, Kelly BT, Voos JE, et al. Surgical technique and anatomic study of latissimus dorsi and teres major transfers. J Bone Joint Surg Am. 2006;88(7):1524–31.
15. Tauber M, Moursy M, Forstner R, et al. Latissimus dorsi tendon transfer for irreparable rotator cuff tears: a modified technique to improve tendon transfer integrity: surgical technique. J Bone Joint Surg Am. 2010;92(Suppl 1 Pt 2):226–39.
16. Valenti P, Kalouche I, Diaz LC, et al. Results of latissimus dorsi tendon transfer in primary or salvage reconstruction of irreparable rotator cuff tears. Orthop Traumatol Surg Res. 2010;96(2):133–8.
17. Miniaci A, MacLeod M. Transfer of the latissimus dorsi muscle after failed repair of a massive tear of the rotator cuff. A two to five-year review. J Bone Joint Surg Am. 1999;81(8):1120–7.
18. Pearle AD, Voos JE, Kelly BT, et al. Surgical technique and anatomic study of latissimus dorsi and teres major transfers. Surgical technique. J Bone Joint Surg Am. 2007;89(Suppl 2 Pt 2):284–96.
19. Goutallier D, Postel JM, Bernageau J, et al. Fatty muscle degeneration in cuff ruptures. Pre- and postoperative evaluation by CT scan. Clin Orthop Relat Res. 1994;(304):78–83.
20. Werner CM, Zingg PO, Lie D, et al. The biomechanical role of the subscapularis in latissimus dorsi transfer for the treatment of irreparable rotator cuff tears. J Shoulder Elbow Surg. 2006;15(6):736–42.
21. Longo UG, Franceschetti E, Petrillo S, et al. Latissimus dorsi tendon transfer for massive irreparable rotator cuff tears: a systematic review. Sports Med Arthrosc. 2011;19(4):428–37.
22. Aoki M, Okamura K, Fukushima S, et al. Transfer of latissimus dorsi for irreparable rotator-cuff tears. J Bone Joint Surg Br. 1996;78(5):761–6.
23. Boileau P, Chuinard C, Roussanne Y, et al. Reverse shoulder arthroplasty combined with a modified latissimus dorsi and teres major tendon transfer for shoulder pseudoparalysis associated with dropping arm. Clin Orthop Relat Res. 2008;466(3):584–93.

24. Iannotti JP, Hennigan S, Herzog R, et al. Latissimus dorsi tendon transfer for irreparable posterosuperior rotator cuff tears. Factors affecting outcome. J Bone Joint Surg Am. 2006;88(2):342–8.

25. Irlenbusch U, Bernsdorf M, Born S, et al. Electromyographic analysis of muscle function after latissimus dorsi tendon transfer. J Shoulder Elbow Surg. 2008;17(3):492–9.

26. Warner JJ, Parsons 4th IM. Latissimus dorsi tendon transfer: a comparative analysis of primary and salvage reconstruction of massive, irreparable rotator cuff tears. J Shoulder Elbow Surg. 2001;10(6):514–21.

27. Weening AA, Willems WJ. Latissimus dorsi transfer for treatment of irreparable rotator cuff tears. Int Orthop. 2010;34(8):1239–44.

28. Costouros JG, Espinosa N, Schmid MR, et al. Teres minor integrity predicts outcome of latissimus dorsi tendon transfer for irreparable rotator cuff tears. J Shoulder Elbow Surg. 2007;16(6):727–34.

29. Debeer P, De Smet L. Outcome of latissimus dorsi transfer for irreparable rotator cuff tears. Acta Orthop Belg. 2010;76(4):449–55.

30. Gerhardt C, Lehmann L, Lichtenberg S, et al. Modified L'Episcopo tendon transfers for irreparable rotator cuff tears: 5-year follow-up. Clin Orthop Relat Res. 2010;468(6):1572–7.

31. Birmingham PM, Neviaser RJ. Outcome of latissimus dorsi transfer as a salvage procedure for failed rotator cuff repair with loss of elevation. J Shoulder Elbow Surg. 2008;17(6):871–4.

Pectoralis Major Tendon Transfer

8

Jeffrey D. Boatright, Austin J. Crow,
and Stephen F. Brockmeier

Pearls and Pitfalls

Pearls

- In the setting of massive superior rotator cuff tears always have a high index of suspicion that the subscapularis may also be involved. The belly-press and lift-off tests are useful tools to aid in diagnosis.
- Indications for pectoralis major tendon transfer are pain or dysfunction arising from an irreparable subscapularis tear, either isolated with an intact superior rotator cuff or in association with a reparable supraspinatus tear. Transfer is also considered in patients with subscapularis insufficiency associated with dynamic anterior instability after a failed prior open stabilization procedure.
- The musculocutaneous nerve must be identified beneath the conjoined tendon; it generally runs 5 cm distal to the tip of the coracoid process.
- If performing a subcoracoid transfer, it is important to check the musculocutaneous nerve after the pectoralis major has been passed to ensure it is not under tension. If it is under tension, the muscle belly can be debulked or a supracoracoid transfer can be carried out.
- In the setting of anterior instability with an irreparable subscapularis tear, it may be beneficial to also perform a labral repair and capsulorrhaphy.

Pitfalls

- Contraindications for pectoralis major tendon transfer include advanced patient age (>65), glenohumeral joint arthrosis, a concomitant irreparable superior rotator cuff tear, fixed anterior joint subluxation, and an inability to comply with postoperative measures and rehabilitation.
- Pectoralis major tendon transfer may not be a good option in the setting of subscapularis repair failure after total shoulder arthroplasty.

J.D. Boatright, MD, MS
Department of Orthopaedic Surgery, University of Virginia Medical Center, University of Virginia, P.O. Box 801016, Charlottesville, VA 22908, USA
e-mail: JB9CT@hscmail.mcc.virginia.edu

A.J. Crow, MD
Department of Orthopedic Surgery, University of Virginia, P.O. Box 801016, Charlottesville, VA 22908, USA
e-mail: AJC9V@hscmail.mcc.virginia.edu

S.F. Brockmeier, MD (✉)
Department of Orthopedic Surgery, University of Virginia, 400 Ray C. Hunt Drive, Suite 300, Charlottesville, VA 22908, USA
e-mail: SFB2E@hscmail.mcc.virginia.edu

L.V. Gulotta and E.V. Craig (eds.), *Massive Rotator Cuff Tears: Diagnosis and Management*,
DOI 10.1007/978-1-4899-7494-5_8, © Springer Science+Business Media New York 2015

- Injury to the lateral pectoral nerve can occur if the pectoralis major is mobilized more than 8 cm.
- Aggressive retraction of the conjoined tendon can result in traction injury to the musculocutaneous nerve.

Introduction

Rotator cuff disease is one of the most prevalent musculoskeletal disorders treated by orthopedic surgeons. Most frequently, this pathology involves the supraspinatus tendon; however, tears of the subscapularis occur commonly, comprising between 3.5 and 8 % of all rotator cuff tears [1–3], with evidence that such tears frequently go undiagnosed [4, 5]. Normal shoulder biomechanics depend heavily upon a properly functioning rotator cuff to provide dynamic stability to the glenohumeral joint. Subscapularis tears have a variable clinical presentation with the more common findings being anterior shoulder pain, weakness with humeral internal rotation, increased passive external rotation, and less frequently anterior glenohumeral instability. There is often a substantial delay in diagnosis, especially in the setting of isolated subscapularis injuries, due to the more subtle presentation [2, 6, 7].

The majority of subscapularis tears can be treated with either arthroscopic or open primary repair. Significant fatty infiltration, muscular atrophy, tendon retraction, and large tear size all make primary repair less likely to succeed and, if severe enough, make a subscapularis tear irreparable [8–11]. The management of an irreparable subscapularis tear can present a significant challenge with musculotendinous transfer of the pectoralis major being the most common treatment option employed.

In this chapter we will review the epidemiology of subscapularis tears, relevant anatomy and biomechanics of the shoulder, and the pathophysiology of subscapularis insufficiency. The common history and physical examination of patients presenting with subscapularis pathology will be discussed, including pertinent findings on diagnostic studies and imaging. We will then examine the indications and contraindications for pectoralis major transfer as a treatment option for irreparable subscapularis tears, followed by an overview of the techniques that have been described for this procedure as well as postoperative rehabilitation. Next, we will outline our preferred technique complete with common pearls and pitfalls based upon our experience with pectoralis major transfer as a treatment option for irreparable subscapularis tears. We will conclude by discussing outcomes and complications related to this procedure by examining the orthopedic literature.

Background

Epidemiology

The prevalence of subscapularis tears reported in the literature varies widely with the most frequently quoted data suggesting that such tears comprise between 3.5 and 8 % of all rotator cuff pathology [1–3]. The vast majority of these tears are reparable, either by arthroscopic or open means. There is essentially no meaningful data regarding the prevalence of irreparable subscapularis tears, most likely due to the relative infrequent nature of such tears and a lack of consistency in defining this lesion. The mean age of patients undergoing pectoralis major transfer for irreparable subscapularis tears in the literature ranges from 49 to 67 years, with males being significantly more likely to undergo this procedure [12–18].

Some of the original investigations regarding the prevalence of subscapularis tears were autopsy studies that demonstrated a subscapularis tear rate of between 3.5 and 20.8 % [1, 19]. In a large MRI study of patients with known rotator cuff tears, the subscapularis tendon was involved approximately 2 % of the time, with 27 % of these being partial thickness tears and 73 % being full-thickness tears [20]. The reason for this variable data is likely multifactorial. Subscapularis tears frequently go undiagnosed, making their true prevalence difficult to accurately report. Recent literature has revealed that difficulty in visualizing subscapularis tears both on MRI and intraoperatively has resulted in significant underestimation of their true prevalence [4, 5]. The advancement of arthroscopy has allowed recognition of previously undiagnosed subscapularis tears with some more recent studies reporting subscapularis involvement in approximately 30 % of all shoulder arthroscopic procedures and between 40 and 59 % of all arthroscopic rotator cuff repairs [4, 21–23]. It must be noted that the large majority of these tears were partial articular-sided tears, the clinical significance of which is still highly debated.

Subscapularis tears are heterogenous in their etiology and clinical presentation. They may be traumatic in nature [2, 6], associated with recurrent anterior glenohumeral dislocations [24–26], or degenerative in nature. They can occur as either isolated lesions, or, more commonly, as a part of a larger tear involving other tendons of the rotator cuff. When subscapularis tears do occur, they are far more likely to occur in association with tears of the supraspinatus than as isolated lesions. In a review of 348 consecutive arthroscopic rotator cuff repairs, Garavaglia et al. reported that 89 % involved the supraspinatus, 37 % involved the subscapularis, and 14 % involved the infraspinatus, with only 1.4 % having an isolated subscapularis tear [27]. In a recent study of 51 patients undergoing arthroscopic subscapularis repair by Lanz et al., 13 % were isolated subscapularis ruptures, 37 % had both subscapularis and supraspinatus involvement, and 50 % involved the subscapularis, supraspinatus, and infraspinatus tendons [28].

Further complicating the mixed epidemiological data is the fact that there is frequently a substantial delay in diagnosis [2, 6, 7]. In a study of 14 traumatic subscapularis tears, Gerber and Krushell [6] found that only 3 were diagnosed soon after the injury with the remaining 11 having a delay in diagnosis that averaged 18 months (range 7–38 months). These lesions are often initially misdiagnosed as subacromial impingement, muscle strain, and long head of the biceps tendon pathology. While much less common,

there is data to suggest that severe isolated subscapularis tears tend to occur at a higher frequency in younger males and are more likely to be associated with anterior instability, which is frequently of a traumatic etiology [2, 6, 12, 29, 30]. In a study by Elhassan et al. involving patients undergoing pectoralis major transfer for irreparable subscapularis repairs, those undergoing the procedure as a result of failed anterior instability surgery had a mean age of 37 versus those undergoing the procedure for other reasons where the mean age was 57 [12].

Anatomy, Biomechanics, and Pathophysiology of Subscapularis Insufficiency

In order to understand pectoralis major transfer as a treatment option for irreparable subscapularis tears, one must have an understanding of the relevant shoulder anatomy, normal shoulder biomechanics, and the pathophysiology of subscapularis insufficiency. The primary function of the subscapularis muscle is internal rotation of the humerus. The pectoralis major, teres major, and latissimus dorsi are partially synergistic with the subscapularis in this function. It is this synergism in conjunction with relative location and similar (though certainly not identical) force vectors of the pectoralis major that serves as the basis for pectoralis major tendon transfer as a treatment option for irreparable subscapularis tears. The subscapularis muscle also plays a role in flexion, extension, adduction, and abduction of the shoulder depending upon the position of the arm [31]. Perhaps more important than the abovementioned functions is the role of the subscapularis in the balanced force couples about the glenohumeral joint, providing dynamic stability to the joint through functional shoulder range of motion.

The subscapularis has the largest cross-sectional area and is the most powerful of all rotator cuff muscles, generating over 50 % of the total power of the rotator cuff [32]. It originates from the anterior surface of the scapula, and as it courses laterally, it travels beneath the coracoid process with the musculotendinous transition point occurring at approximately the level of the glenoid rim. The upper two-thirds of the tendon inserts on the lesser tuberosity with the inferior third inserting on the humeral metaphysis. This forms a trapezoidal-shaped footprint that measures approximately 2.5 cm in the superior-inferior dimension [33].

The superior aspect of the subscapularis forms the inferior border of the rotator interval, a triangular space located in the anterosuperior aspect of the glenohumeral joint. The base of the rotator interval is formed medially at the level of the coracoid process, with the apex laterally defined by the transverse humeral ligament, and the superior border formed by the inferior margin of the supraspinatus. The rotator interval has classically been described as containing the coracohumeral ligament, superior glenohumeral ligament, long head of the biceps tendon, and the glenohumeral capsule.

The subscapularis in conjunction with the coracohumeral ligament and superior glenohumeral ligament forms the biceps pulley mechanism which has been shown to be critical for biceps tendon stability within the glenohumeral joint and in the bicipital groove. This relationship explains the association between the often seen concurrent subscapularis and biceps tendon pathology. Subscapularis tears can lead to improper tensioning of the biceps pulley leading to subluxation or frank dislocation of the biceps tendon from the bicipital groove. It also partially explains the well-documented delay in diagnosis in patients with subscapularis tears and anterior shoulder pain that is sometimes initially misattributed to isolated biceps tendon pathology [6].

The subscapularis is innervated by the upper and lower subscapular nerves both of which typically branch from the posterior cord of the brachial plexus and are derived from C5 and C6 nerve fibers. There is more anatomic variation with the lower subscapular nerve. It occasionally branches from the origin of the axillary nerve or from the thoracodorsal nerve itself and may also contain C7 nerve fibers [34].

The glenohumeral joint allows for greater range of motion than any other joint in the human body. This range of motion is afforded, in large part, at the direct expense of decreased joint stability. For this reason, a properly functioning shoulder must achieve a fine balance between mobility and stability, which is the product of a complex set of biomechanical interactions between the static and dynamic stabilizers about the glenohumeral joint.

The static stabilizers can be further subdivided into bony and soft tissue stabilizers. Bony static stabilizers include the glenoid and humeral head and the degree of articular congruence between these two structures. The glenoid is often described as pear shaped being 20 % larger inferiorly than it is superiorly. It has a surface area that is roughly one-third that of the humeral head and has a radius of curvature mismatch of +2.3 mm (approx. 10 %) compared to the radius of curvature of the humeral head in the coronal plane [35]. This data emphasizes the importance of the soft tissue stabilizers to the overall stability of the glenohumeral joint. Static soft tissue stabilizers consist of the glenohumeral ligaments, glenohumeral capsule, glenoid labrum, and the negative intra-articular pressure with the joint. All have been shown to play a role in glenohumeral stability.

Perhaps the most important structures to the overall stability of the glenohumeral joint during physiologic range of motion are the dynamic soft tissue stabilizers. These include the muscles of the rotator cuff (subscapularis, supraspinatus, infraspinatus, teres minor), the deltoid, the long head of the biceps, and to a lesser extent the other periscapular muscles including the latissimus dorsi, teres major, and the pectoralis major.

The rotator cuff muscles play a crucial role in the balanced force couples about the glenohumeral joint which are essential for normal shoulder biomechanics, and some argue this to be the most important role of the subscapularis [36–41]. These balanced force couples help establish equilibrium within the joint and must be maintained for any given arm position. The subscapularis plays a vital role in this balance in both the coronal and transverse planes [36, 37]. During normal shoulder abduction the superior moment of the deltoid is balanced by the inferomedial moment

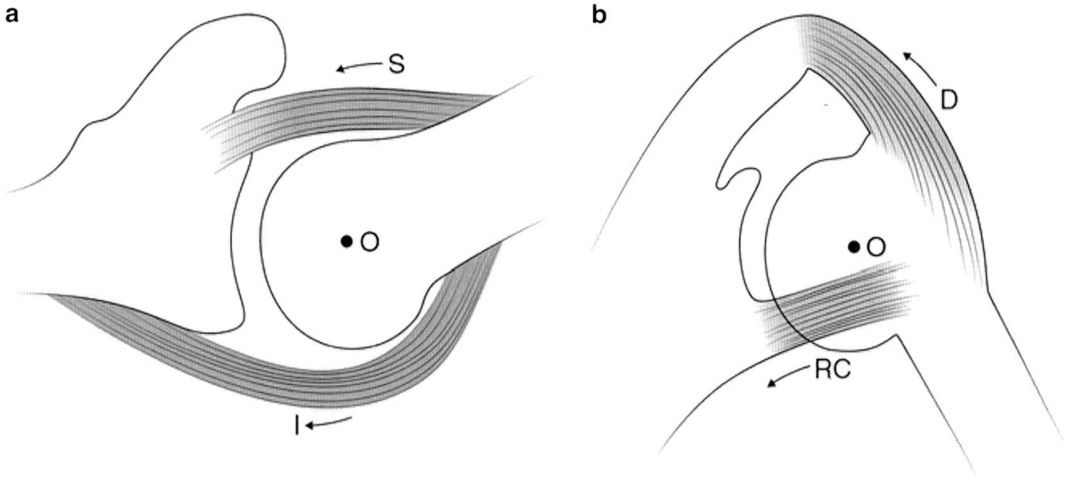

a

b

Fig. 8.1 Force couples about the glenohumeral joint. (a) The transverse plane force couple consists of the opposing moments created between the subscapularis (*S*) anteriorly and the combined moment of the infraspinatus and teres minor (*I*) posteriorly. (b) The coronal place force couple. The superior moment of the deltoid (*D*) is balanced by the inferomedial moment of the inferior rotator cuff (*RC*) that is provided by the sum of the individual moments of the subscapularis, infraspinatus, and teres minor with a line of action that is inferior to the center of rotation of the humeral head (*O*) (Reprinted from Omid and Lee [58], with permission. ©2013 American Academy of Orthopaedic Surgeons)

of the inferior rotator cuff that is provided by the sum of the individual moments of the subscapularis, infraspinatus, and teres minor with a line of action that is inferior to the center of rotation of the humeral head [40] (Fig. 8.1b). This coronal plane force couple must be maintained throughout the range of motion in order to create a stable fulcrum within the glenohumeral joint. This is essential for stable and efficient shoulder elevation. Burkhart utilized fluoroscopic imaging to demonstrate that massive rotator cuff tears involving the subscapularis failed to maintain this force couple resulting in an unstable fulcrum leading to anterosuperior humeral head translation during shoulder abduction [37]. Further illustrating the importance of the subscapularis in this force couple, Thompson et al. demonstrated a stable fulcrum with normal humeral head translation in a cadaveric model with supraspinatus tears up to 5 cm as long as subscapularis and infraspinatus function was intact [41].

The subscapularis plays a crucial role in the transverse plane force couple as well. The transverse plane force couple consists of the opposing moments created between the subscapularis anteriorly and the combined moment of the infraspinatus and teres minor posteriorly (Fig. 8.1a). A stable force couple in the transverse plane provides concavity compression providing stability and preventing anterior-posterior translation of the humeral head within the glenoid [36]. This stabilizing effect is supported by a recent EMG study in which David et al. demonstrated that the rotator cuff muscles are activated prior to the deltoid and other periscapular muscles in normal shoulder motion, suggesting a need to provide concavity compression and stabilization prior to initiating glenohumeral motion [38].

History and Presentation

The clinical presentation of patients with a subscapularis tear can be quite variable, depending largely upon the etiology and chronicity of the injury. In the case of an acute traumatic subscapularis tear, the patient will often report a traumatic external rotation and/or hyperextension force with the arm in an adducted position, with nearly half of these being sports related [2, 6]. Nearly all of these patients will report anterior shoulder pain with activities of daily living both above and below the level of the shoulder and weakness in the affected shoulder. Seventy percent will have anterior shoulder night pain, and 50 % will report inability to work secondary to their pain [2].

In the majority of patients, a subscapularis tear will present in the setting of a massive rotator cuff tear with concurrent involvement of the supraspinatus and possibly infraspinatus tendons as well. These are often chronic and degenerative in nature and will often present with a constellation of symptoms indistinguishable from that of a standard rotator cuff tear.

Another subset of patients with subscapularis tears will have experienced recurrent anterior shoulder dislocations; thus, it is important to ascertain this history during the clinical interview as well. It is important to maintain a high level of suspicion for subscapularis tendon involvement in each of these subsets of patients as it has been shown that there is often a significant delay in diagnosis resulting in interval degeneration, atrophy, fatty infiltration, and tendon retraction, all of which have direct implications on the reparability of the tear and overall outcome [8–11].

Clinical Examination

As with any orthopedic physical examination, evaluation of the shoulder in a patient with suspected subscapularis disease should proceed in a logical, organized, and efficient manner directed at elucidating the underlying pathology. It should always include a comparison to the contralateral side. It should proceed through inspection, palpation, assessment of both passive and active range of motion, and assessment of joint stability, followed by strength and provocative testing.

As stated previously, patients with subscapularis tears will frequently have anterior shoulder pain that worsens with activity both above and below the level of the shoulder; however, this is neither sensitive nor specific for subscapularis pathology. Patients with a subscapularis tear associated with recurrent glenohumeral instability will be expected to have physical examination findings consistent with instability such as a

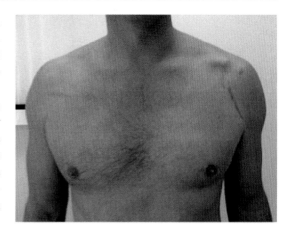

Fig. 8.2 Clinical photograph of a patient with a left-sided irreparable subscapularis tear. Note the anterior shoulder musculature atrophy on the affected side as well as the prior surgical incision. This patient had failed a prior attempt at open primary repair

positive apprehension and Jobe relocation test and possibly a positive sulcus sign. Additionally, when examining a patient with shoulder complaints, the examining physician must also consider the possibility of cervical spine disease manifesting as shoulder pain and/or weakness. The patient should be examined in a gown with both shoulders exposed. Inspection may reveal atrophy of the anterior shoulder with asymmetry to the contralateral side. Prior surgical incisions should be noted (Fig. 8.2). Scapular mechanics with elevation and abduction should be noted with attention to any dyskinesis, winging, or compensatory scapular motion patterns. Palpation of the lesser tuberosity or bicipital groove may elicit pain in the setting of subscapularis injury with or without biceps involvement.

The majority of physical examination tests directed at evaluating a possible subscapularis tear come in the form of range of motion and strength testing. Frequently patients with a complete subscapularis tear will exhibit increased passive external rotation compared to the contralateral shoulder [6]. Loss of the integrity of the subscapularis as a restraint to excessive external rotation is responsible for this finding, and this may be subtle or nonexistent in partial tears or in patients with concurrent degenerative conditions.

A number of specific examination tests have been described to assess subscapularis integrity. The most common of these tests are the lift-off

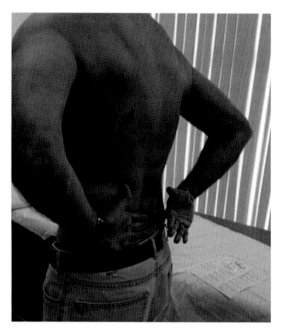

Fig. 8.3 Clinical photograph of the lift-off test on a patient with a left-sided irreparable subscapularis tear. The patient demonstrates a positive lift-off test on the left suggesting weakness of the subscapularis as the primary internal rotator of the humerus

test, internal rotation lag test, the belly-off sign, an[6, 22, 42–46]. The lift-off te and Krushell [6] evaluate placing the dorsum of the affected shoulder onto the and asking the patient to the back in a posterior di nally rotating the arm. the patient's inability to ness of the subscapulari rotator of the humerus rotation lag sign descri begins with the patient examining physician and the dorsum of the nally rotating the arm the patient's back. Th maintain this position the hand. The test is patient is unable to (Fig. 8.4). Multiple va test have been describe this test is performed both hands flat on the close to the body in 9 patient is then asked to men while bringing the

he belly-press ar-hug test [6, bed by Gerber bscapularis by the side of the 's lumbar spine lift the hand off by further inter- e test indicates suggests weak- primary internal .3). The internal Hertel et al. [44] lar position. The bilizes the elbow while further inter- ng the hand off of nt is then asked to e examiner releases dered positive if the intain this position ons of the belly-press 2, 47, 48]. In general, aving the patient place domen with the elbow degrees of flexion. The press in against the abdo- elbow forward while

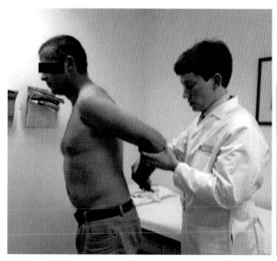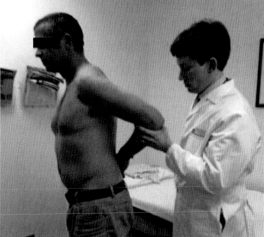

Fig. 8.4 Clinical photograph of the internal rotation lag sign. The patient demonstrates a positive internal rotation lag sign by his inability to maintain the position of his hand when the examining physician releases it

maintaining a straightened posture of the wrist (Fig. 8.5). Depending on the variation used, the test can be considered positive if there is (1) asymmetry in the amount of anterior movement of the elbow (less forward movement indicating subscapularis weakness), (2) less posteriorly directed force into the abdomen (as measured by a tensiometer), (3) clinical evidence of elbow and or shoulder extension while performing the maneuver (as compensation for subscapularis weakness), or (4) differences in the wrist flexion angle at the terminus of the maneuver (as measured by a goniometer, with the pathologic side showing greater wrist flexion). This final variation has been described as the Napoleon sign, named as such based upon the position in which Napoleon Bonaparte held his hand in multiple portraits [49, 50]. The belly-off sign, described by Scheibel et al. [46], begins with the patient in a similar position to that of the belly-press test. The examiner then supports the elbow with one hand and brings it into a position of maximum internal rotation by bringing the elbow forward while stabilizing the palm of the patient's hand against the abdomen. The examiner then asks the

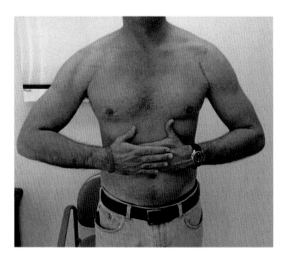

Fig. 8.5 Clinical photograph of the belly-press test on a patient with a left-sided irreparable subscapularis tear. The patient demonstrates a positive belly-press test on the left. Notice the asymmetry in the amount of anterior translation of the elbow (R > L). Again note the difference in anterior shoulder muscle tone and prior surgical incision on the left

patient to actively maintain that position while releasing the patient's hand. An inability to maintain the palm against the abdomen, or wrist flexion as a compensatory mechanism, constitutes a positive test. The bear-hug test, described by Barth et al. [22], is performed by placing the palm of the affected shoulder on the contralateral shoulder with the elbow pointed anteriorly and the humerus in 90 degrees of forward flexion. The examiner applies an external rotation force to the arm by attempting to lift the hand off the shoulder while asking the patient to actively resist this force. An inability to resist this force implies subscapularis weakness and thus constitutes a positive test (Fig. 8.6).

Numerous studies have evaluated the diagnostic value of these clinical tests. In an electromyographic study, Pennock et al. [45] evaluated the effect of arm and shoulder position on isolating the subscapularis from the remainder of the cuff musculature as well as differential activation of the upper and lower subscapularis while performing the bear-hug, belly-press, and lift-off tests. They concluded that the level of subscapularis activation was similar for all three tests regardless of arm position, with each being significantly greater than that of the other rotator cuff muscles. Furthermore, they found that shoulder and arm positioning did not produce significantly different results between the upper and lower divisions of the subscapularis within and between each of the three tests. Bartsch et al. [51] examined 50 consecutive patients who were scheduled to undergo shoulder arthroscopy, subjecting them to the lift-off test, internal rotation lag sign, belly-press test, and belly-off test. The clinical exams were then compared to the arthroscopic findings. They concluded that the most sensitive tests were the belly-press test and belly-off tests (88 % and 87 %, respectively), the most specific test was the belly-off test (91 %), and the most accurate test being the belly-off test (90 %). Fifteen percent of subscapularis tears were not detected by any of the aforementioned tests, although it is worth noting that the majority of the tears in this study were partial thickness in nature. Rigsby et al. [52] performed a systematic review of the available literature from which pooled indices regarding

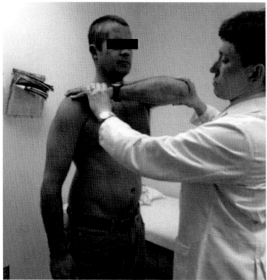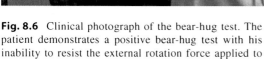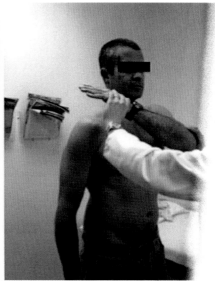

Fig. 8.6 Clinical photograph of the bear-hug test. The patient demonstrates a positive bear-hug test with his inability to resist the external rotation force applied to his shoulder which is imparted by the [exami]ng physician by lifting the patient's hand off [the con]tralateral shoulder

the diagnostic value of the lift-off test, internal rotation lag sign, Napoleon sign, bear-hug test, belly-off test, and belly-press test were developed specifically as they relate to full-thickness subscapularis tears. They concluded that the Napoleon sign (sensitivity 98 %, specificity 97 %), internal rotation lag sign (sensitivity 98 %, specificity 94 %), and lift-off test (sensitivity 94 %, specificity 99 %) were all clinically useful tests for ruling in and ruling out full-thickness subscapularis tears. There is no literature examining the diagnostic value of these physical examination findings as they relate to irreparable subscapularis tears.

Imaging

As with most orthopedic evaluations, imaging studies often start with plain radiographs. Three views, including an AP in the scapular plane, an axillary lateral, and a scapular-Y, should be obtained and are generally normal in patients with subscapularis tears. Chronic tears, especially those associated with anterior glenohumeral instability, may demonstrate anterior subluxation on the axillary lateral radiographs, but this is neither sensitive n[or spe]cific for a subscapularis tear. In patients w[ith ma]ssive rotator cuff tears, which sometime[s inclu]de the subscapularis, one may see a hig[h-ridi]ng humeral head relative to the glenoid and [narr]owing of the acromiohumeral space. In pati[ents] with chronic massive rotator cuff tears, ther[e ma]y be degenerative changes noted on plain ra[dio]graphs such as joint space narrowing, subch[on]dral sclerosis, rimming inferior osteophytes, [a]nd potentially signs of rotator cuff tear arthropathy such as superior glenoid wear and acetabularization of the undersurface of the acromion.

Ultrasound has increased in popularity as an imaging modality for visualizing the rotator cuff and diagnosing related pathology. It is relatively inexpensive, noninvasive, and allows for easy comparison to the contralateral shoulder. Teefey et al. evaluated the accuracy of ultrasound compared to arthroscopy in detecting rotator cuff lesions and reported 100 % sensitivity and 85 % specificity in detecting all rotator cuff tears, and accurately diagnosed 6 of 7 subscapularis tears [53]. These results approach those reported by MRI; however, the ability to accurately quantify the size and depth of partial-thickness tears as well as the ability to distinguish between partial- and

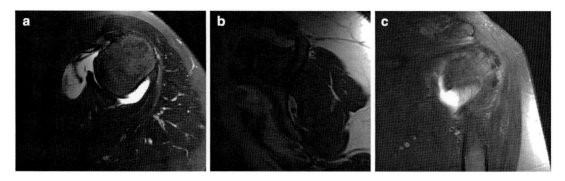

Fig. 8.7 (a) Axial MRI arthrography of a patient with a subscapularis tear. Note the wispy, disorganized tendon morphology, absence of a clear subscapularis tendon footprint, medial subluxation of the biceps tendon, and substantial retraction of the subscapularis muscle belly. (b) Sagittal MRI of a patient with a subscapularis tear. Note the substantial muscle atrophy and Goutallier stage 4 fatty infiltration. (c) Coronal MRI arthrography of a patient with a subscapularis tear. Note the detachment of the tendon from its insertion on the lesser tuberosity, significant fraying, and consequent uncovering of the anterior humeral head with medial retraction of the muscle belly

full-thickness tears is often called into question; thus the role in ultrasound as a routine imaging modality for diagnosing rotator cuff pathology remains undefined.

MRI is the imaging modality of choice for diagnosing and characterizing rotator cuff tears, including those of the subscapularis. CT arthrogram can be utilized in those unable to undergo MRI. MRI arthrography has been shown to be superior to standard MRI for the diagnosis of rotator cuff tears [54] as has fat-saturated imaging versus standard sequences [55]. Abnormally high signal in the subscapularis tendon on T2-weighted imaging, disorganized tendon morphology, frank disruption of the subscapularis tendon, contrast leakage onto the lesser tuberosity during arthrography, subscapularis muscle belly atrophy and/or fatty infiltration, and medial subluxation of the biceps tendon from the bicipital groove are all well-accepted MRI findings that should alert the physician as to a possible subscapularis tear (Fig. 8.7a–c). In a study on traumatic tears of the subscapularis, Deutsch et al. reported medial subluxation of the biceps tendon on MRI in 46 % of full-thickness tears [2]. A recent study, Jung et al. [56], described a new MRI arthrography finding, coined the "bridging sign," that was highly correlated with full-thickness tears of the subscapularis that also involved at least the anterior half of the supraspinatus. This sign is described as a band-like structure on axial cuts of low to intermediate signal intensity on all sequences that connects the superior margin of the subscapularis to the inferior margin of the supraspinatus through the subcoracoid and subacromial space. It is thought to be the MRI correlate to the arthroscopic "comma sign" as described by Burkhart et al. [49]. For full-thickness subscapularis tears that also involved the anterior half of the subscapularis, the bridging sign was found to have 81 % sensitivity, 100 % specificity, and 86.2 % accuracy [56].

Unlike physical examination and plain radiography, MRI lends critical information regarding the status of the torn tendon and whether it is a repairable injury or likely to require a salvage procedure. While the true and definitive determination of the reparability of a subscapularis tear occurs with intraoperative assessment, advanced imaging studies such as MRI often shed considerable light on the subject preoperatively, allowing the surgeon to begin planning accordingly. No consensus exists regarding what constitutes an irreparable subscapularis tear on MRI; however, some general concepts are routinely applied. Muscle belly atrophy, fatty infiltration, tear size, and degree of tendon retraction have all been shown to be associated with worse clinical outcomes and increased re-tear rates after primary repair of the rotator cuff [8–11]. This has led some surgeons to utilize these findings to various degrees as potential indicators of irreparability. Warner et al. [7] described a grading system to evaluate the amount of subscapularis muscle atrophy on MRI. Their system utilizes T1-weighted sagittal oblique MRI sequences medial to the coracoid process. A line is drawn from the tip of the coracoid process to the inferior tip of the scapular body to define the fossa, and subscapularis muscle belly atrophy is graded as follows: (1) no atrophy – muscle belly fills the fossa and the outer contour is convex in nature; (2) minimal atrophy – muscle belly outer contour is flat with respect to the fossa; (3) moderate atrophy – muscle belly outer contour is concave and does not completely fill the fossa; and (4) severe atrophy – muscle belly is barely evident in the fossa.

Goutallier et al. [8] first described a staging system utilizing axial CT scan to characterize the degree of rotator cuff fatty infiltration. This was divided into five stages: stage 0 – indicating normal muscle; stage 1 – muscle has some fatty streaks; stage 2 – fatty infiltration is important, but more muscle than fat; stage 3 – as much fat as muscle; and stage 4 – more fat than muscle is present. This staging system was later adapted for MRI by Fuchs et al. who evaluated fatty infiltration in the same manner using the most lateral parasagittal MRI cut in which the scapular spine is attached to the scapular body [57]. The evaluation of subscapularis tendon retraction is relatively straightforward and best evaluated on axial imaging. Most of the literature regarding irreparable subscapularis tears utilizes MRI characteristics as inclusion criteria. Generally speaking, subscapularis tears with Goutallier stage 3 or 4, fatty infiltration, and ± subscapularis tendon retraction to the level of glenoid rim are considered irreparable [8–11, 58]. As stated previously, the definitive and final determination of subscapularis reparability is determined intraoperatively.

Indications and Contraindications for Pectoralis Major Transfer for Subscapularis Insufficiency

Pectoralis major transfer for an irreparable anterosuperior rotator cuff tear was first described by Wirth and Rockwood in 1997 [18]. Wirth and Rockwood's original indications for pectoralis

major transfer were patients with recurren anterior instability in the setting of an irreparab subscapularis tear [18]. Pectoralis major transf has since been reported by multiple authors a treatment of irreparable anterosuperior rota cuff tears [13, 17, 18]. Several modifications the original technique have subsequently be described, with no study to show the superio of one method over the others. The indicati always include an irreparable subscapularis and generally have either anterior instability 18] or significant functional limitations and as features precipitating surgical interve [17, 59]. Pectoralis major transfers have performed in patients with isolated subscap ruptures and those with a concomitant sup natus tear; several studies have shown that fers in the setting of both subscapulari supraspinatus tears have inferior outcome compared to isolated irreparable subsca ruptures [15]. This has led some authors t sider irreparable subscapularis tears in the of an irreparable supraspinatus tear to be tive contraindication to pectoralis major t er [15]. Other contraindications include adv ed patient age (>65), glenohumeral joint art sis, fixed anterior joint subluxation, an inabi y to comply with postoperative measures and rehabilitation, and obviously pectoralis major dysfunction or insufficiency.

The initial management of a massive rotator cuff tear should be a nonsurgical, multifaceted approach. Formal physical therapy, aimed at deltoid and periscapular strengthening, is a key component [60]. Nonsteroidal anti-inflammatories should be used in patients without a contraindication. Corticosteroid injections into the subacromial space or glenohumeral joint can be an adjunct, especially in conjunction with physical therapy.

If nonoperative management has failed, it is first important to differentiate between a "massive" and an "irreparable" rotator cuff repair as these terms are often mistakenly used interchangeably. Not all massive tears are irreparable and several classification systems have been described to help surgeons determine which of these larger tears will be ultimately reparable. Cofield et al. originally classified rotator cuff tears based solely on size, with massive tears being greater than 5 cm in diameter [61]. Gerber later identified massive tears as those involving two or more tendons [62]. The pragmatic definition of an irreparable rotator cuff tear is one where the quality and/or mobility of the tendon does not allow for direct repair to bone. This further differentiation to an irreparable tear is more difficult and generally related to three factors: retraction, atrophy, and fatty infiltration. Goutallier et al. attempted to quantify fatty infiltration by classifying the rotator cuff muscle based on CT findings [8]. The authors also noted a direct correlation between the amount of fatty infiltration and muscular atrophy. Multiple studies have validated the use of the Goutallier classification in MRI studies [57]. The exact cutoff for the amount of fatty infiltration before a rotator cuff tear is irreparable is unknown, but many authors believe Goutallier stage 3 or 4 (50 % or greater fatty infiltration) suggests an irreparable tear [58]. Acromiohumeral distance, measured on plain radiographs of the shoulder, can also be a tool in determining if a RCT is repairable. It has been noted that an acromiohumeral distance of less than 7 mm is suggestive of an irreparable tear [63].

Several other surgical treatment options are available for patients with massive rotator cuff tears including debridement or partial rotator cuff repair. Debridement alone will only offer improvement in pain and no strength or functional improvement, and the durability of this pain relief is thought to be limited [64]. Burkhart et al. found that partial rotator cuff repair can provide improvements in both pain and function [65]. The obvious prerequisite for this option is having some of the rotator cuff muscle and tendon amenable for partial repair; in the setting of a ruptured subscapularis with significant atrophy and fatty infiltration, this is not always possible. In patients who present with chronic anterior-superior instability, reconstruction of the coracoacromial arch has been described, but results have been unsatisfactory in the majority of patients [66]. Another option, in lower demand and more elderly patients, is reverse total shoulder arthroplasty. Early and intermediate outcomes appear promising, but long-term results are not known at this time [67]. For many patients with subscapularis insufficiency, this is not a great option due to age and functional demands.

Technique

Subcoracoid Pectoralis Major Transfer

Subcoracoid pectoralis major transfer, with several variations, has been described by several authors including Resch et al. [17] and Galatz et al. [13]. The surgery is performed under general anesthesia and augmented with a preoperative regional block. The patient is placed into a beach chair position, preferably with a hydraulic/

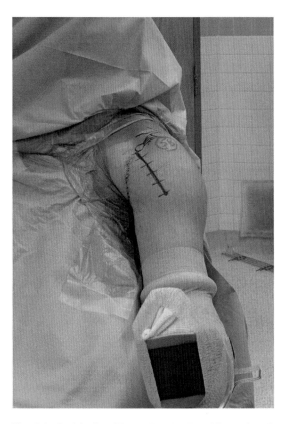

Fig. 8.8 Positioning. The patient is placed into a beach chair position, then prepped and draped in the standard sterile fashion. The arm is placed into a commercially available arm positioner, and bony landmarks are identified. Note the prior surgical scar from an open subscapularis primary repair that ultimately failed

pneumatic arm holder to facilitate easy positioning of the arm intraoperatively (Fig. 8.8); positioning the arm with a padded Mayo stand is an alternative option. After the arm is prepped and draped, a standard deltopectoral approach is used to gain exposure to the anterior shoulder. Care should be taken to avoid violating the deltopectoral fascia until full-thickness skin flaps are mobilized and the fat stripe containing the cephalic vein is identified; this helps to avoid incidental dissection through the deltoid. Once the cephalic vein is identified, it should be mobilized, along with the deltoid, laterally. This will expose the conjoined tendon. A self-retaining retractor can be placed beneath the pectoralis major medially and the deltoid laterally to assist with exposure. The clavipectoral fascia should then be incised just lateral to the conjoined tendon, which will expose the anterior shoulder.

In the setting of an irreparable subscapularis tear, the tendon will be avulsed from its insertion on the lesser tuberosity and retracted medially; in addition, the long head of the biceps will generally either be dislocated medially, partially torn with associated tendon degeneration, or ruptured (Fig. 8.9). If the long head of the biceps is present and does not have significant distal degeneration, biceps tenodesis is generally carried out in the subpectoral position. In the setting of advanced degeneration, a long head biceps tenotomy is preferred.

Next, the conjoined tendon should be further mobilized by blunt dissection. The previously placed self-retaining retractor can be adjusted so it is deep to the deltoid laterally and the conjoined tendon medially. The location of the musculocutaneous nerve can then be identified by palpation, which will generally be 5 cm distal to the coracoid process [68] (Fig. 8.10). Some authors recommend fully dissecting the musculocutaneous nerve [13] while others feel that this is unnecessary [17] and that the transferred pectoralis tendon can be passed in a "blind" fashion.

The pectoralis major tendon is identified at its insertion lateral to the bicipital groove. The desired portion of the muscle and tendon can then be released sharply from the bone. Resch et al. [17] advocate using the superior one-half to two-thirds of the pectoralis major, while Galatz et al. [13]

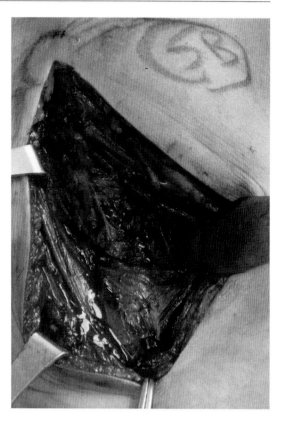

Fig. 8.9 Deltopectoral approach. A standard deltopectoral approach is utilized to gain access to the anterior shoulder. Note the paucity of identifiable subscapularis tendon and complete absence of the long head of the biceps tendon

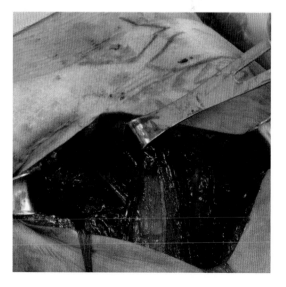

Fig. 8.10 Musculocutaneous nerve. Note the musculocutaneous nerve diving into the undersurface of the conjoint tendon approximately 5 cm distal to the coracoid process

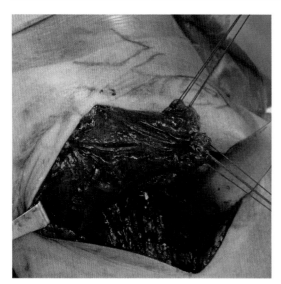

Fig. 8.11 Mobilization of the pectoralis major. The pectoralis major tendon has been released from its insertion lateral to the bicipital groove and mobilized for ease of passage. Stay sutures in the tendon have been placed to facilitate the transfer

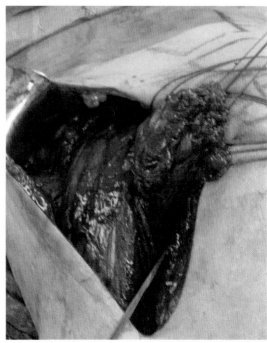

Fig. 8.12 Passage of the pectoralis major musculotendinous unit. The pectoralis major musculotendinous unit is passed posterior to the conjoined tendon and superior/anterior to the musculocutaneous nerve

recommend transfer of the entire musculotendinous unit (Fig. 8.11). It is useful to place several stay sutures in the released tendon to assist with manipulation and passing of the tendon. After the tendon is released, the pectoralis major muscle should be mobilized in preparation for transfer. It is important not to mobilize the muscle more than 8 cm medial to the tendon due to potential injury to the lateral pectoral nerve [69]. The tendon should then be passed posterior to the conjoined tendon and superior/anterior to the musculocutaneous nerve (Fig. 8.12). It is important to assess the nerve once the tendon has been passed, as the large pectoralis major muscle belly can place it under undue tension leading to a risk for neurologic sequelae. If the nerve is felt to be under tension, several options have been proposed including debulking the muscle [17] or release of a small proximal branch of the musculocutaneous nerve to the coracobrachialis while leaving the main innervation to the biceps brachii intact [13]

A grasping stitch, such as a Mason-Allen stitch, should be placed into the tendon with a #2 or larger, braided, nonabsorbable suture. The humerus is prepared by decortication with a

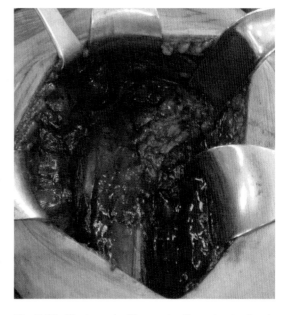

Fig. 8.13 Final repair. The pectoralis major tendon is then repaired to the bone using bone anchors in the anatomic location of the subscapularis tendon insertion along the lateral wall of the bicipital groove

high-speed burr. The tendon is then repaired to the bone with the use of bone anchors or a transosseous technique (Fig. 8.13). The location of repair is somewhat controversial, with descriptions of transfer to the lesser tuberosity [13], both the greater and lesser tuberosity [14, 17], and into the bicipital groove [59] having been described.

The wound is then copiously irrigated with sterile saline and then the incision is closed in layers. Generally, a drain is not necessary, but if meticulous hemostasis is not achieved, then a drain can be placed to prevent formation of a hematoma.

Supracoracoid Pectoralis Major Transfer

Split pectoralis major transfer anterior to the conjoined tendon has been previously described by Warner [59]. The surgery is performed under general anesthesia and augmented with a preoperative regional block. Patient positioning is similar to subcoracoid pectoralis transfer with a hydraulic/pneumatic arm holder used as described above. After the arm is prepped and draped, a standard deltopectoral approach is used to gain exposure to the anterior shoulder. Again, care should be taken to avoid violating the deltopectoral fascia until full-thickness skin flaps are mobilized and the fat stripe containing the cephalic vein is identified to avoid incidental dissection through the deltoid. Once the cephalic vein is identified, it should be mobilized, along with the deltoid, laterally to expose the conjoined tendon. A self-retaining retractor can be placed beneath the pectoralis major medially and the deltoid laterally to assist with exposure. The clavipectoral fascia is then incised just lateral to the conjoined tendon, which will expose the anterior shoulder.

The detached and medially retracted subscapularis is identified and the biceps tendon is evaluated and managed with a tenodesis or tenotomy as delineated above. Repair of the subscapularis should generally be attempted, and with a massive, retracted tear significant mobilization is required. Releasing the subscapularis medially, inferiorly, and superiorly will help the excursion of the tendon. If it can be brought out to the lesser tuberosity, without excess tension, it should be fixed with bone anchors or a transosseous technique. The conjoined tendon should then be further mobilized by blunt dissection, and the location of the musculocutaneous nerve can then be identified by palpation, which will generally be 5 cm distal to the coracoid process [68].

The pectoralis major tendon is identified at its insertion lateral to the bicipital groove. The superior and inferior borders of the pectoralis major are exposed, and the dissection can be taken medially on the superficial surface. If a split transfer is planned, then it is critical to correctly identify the sternal and clavicular heads of the muscle. The sternal head travels partially underneath the clavicular portion which results in a 180 rotation upon its insertion on the humerus [69]. The sternal head can then be released sharply from its insertion on the distal portion of the lateral aspect of the bicipital groove. It is useful to place several stay sutures in the released tendon to assist with manipulation and passing of the tendon. Once the interval between the two heads is identified, it should be bluntly dissected approximately 4–5 cm. The released sternal head is then brought beneath the intact clavicular head.

A grasping stitch, such as a Mason-Allen stitch, should be placed into the tendon with a #2, or larger, braided, nonabsorbable suture. The humerus is then prepared by decortication with a high-speed burr. The tendon is then repaired to the bone with the use of bone anchors or a transosseous technique. The location of repair can be determined based on surgeon's preference, with transfer either to the lesser tuberosity [13], both the greater and lesser tuberosity [14, 17], or into the bicipital groove [59].

The wound is then copiously irrigated with sterile saline and then the incision is closed in layers, with drain placement if necessary to prevent formation of a hematoma.

Postoperative Care and Rehabilitation

There is some variability in the described postoperative treatment, but most authors recommend the shoulder be maintained in an immobilizer between 4 and 6 weeks. Gentle Codman pendulum exercises can be started in the first few days after surgery, either at home or under the care of a physical therapist. The sutures are removed 10–14 days following surgery, and formal physical therapy should be initiated. The first 6 weeks focus on passive and active assisted range of motion. Passive external rotation in adduction and at 45° abduction to the point of initial repair tension as measured intraoperatively can be useful to prevent adhesions of the transferred muscle to the overlying or underlying conjoined tendon.

Some authors [18] advocate strength training once full passive motion is obtained and the patient is 6 weeks from surgery, while others [13, 17, 59] recommend delaying strength training until at least 3 months out from surgery. Because the pectoralis major has a similar function to the subscapularis, biofeedback programs are not as critical to retrain the pectoralis. As with many transfers, improvements in pain and function can be expected up to 1 year out from surgery [58].

Our Preferred Method

At our institution, pectoralis major transfer is the primary salvage option for patients with an irreparable subscapularis tear, either isolated with an intact superior rotator cuff or in association with a reparable supraspinatus tear. Transfer is also considered in patients with subscapularis insufficiency associated with dynamic anterior instability after a failed prior open stabilization procedure. Contraindications for this procedure include advanced patient age (>65), glenohumeral joint arthrosis, a concomitant irreparable superior rotator cuff tear, fixed anterior joint subluxation, and an inability to comply with postoperative measures and rehabilitation. Additionally, based on our experience, pectoralis major transfer has been

an inferior option in the setting of subscapularis repair failure after total shoulder arthroplasty. These patients are managed with either revision subscapularis repair with augmentation or conversion to reverse shoulder arthroplasty.

We prefer a subcoracoid split pectoralis transfer in most patients, similar to the technique described by Resch et al. [17] as described above. Patients are positioned in the beach chair and diagnostic arthroscopy is carried out to confirm an irreparable lesion of the subscapularis and an intact or reparable supraspinatus and infraspinatus. A standard deltopectoral approach is used as delineated previously, and the anterior shoulder and conjoined tendon are exposed. The biceps tendon is tenodesed below the pectoralis using an interference screw. We localize the musculocutaneous nerve but do not generally perform a formal neurolysis. The pectoralis major tendon is then exposed, and the superior ½ of the tendon is released directly from its humeral footprint with placement of multiple stay sutures. After mobilization, the musculotendinous unit is passed deep to the conjoined tendon and fixed to the lesser tuberosity using three suture anchors, with a two medial and one lateral suture bridge technique. Patients are immobilized for 6 weeks in a sling and swathe, with rehab initiating during week 2 with pendulums and passive external rotation in adduction to ~30° to prevent adhesions in the early postoperative period. Active range of motion is initiated at 6 weeks with strengthening beginning at 12 weeks. Patients are counseled that their final functional outcome will not be realized until up to 1 year postsurgery.

Outcomes of Pectoralis Major Tendon Transfer

High-level studies looking at the outcomes of pectoralis major transfers for subscapularis insufficiency are lacking, with a majority of the studies being small series that are retrospective in nature. In addition the indications and inclusion/exclusion criteria are variable between the studies that do look at outcomes. Furthermore, there was considerable variability in the portion of pectoralis transferred, fixation method, and postoperative protocols [12, 13, 15, 17, 18, 59]. In spite of the abovementioned shortcomings, there are several trends in patient outcomes following pectoralis major transfer including improved pain and incremental improvement in function.

Wirth and Rockwood [18] reported on 13 patients, with a mean follow-up of 5 years, with irreparable subscapularis ruptures and recurrent anterior instability following failure of a capsular repair. Seven patients had transfers of the pectoralis major only, while five had transfer of both the pectoralis major and minor, and one had transfer of only the pectoralis minor. On the basis of ASES shoulder scores, ten had satisfactory outcomes, while three had unsatisfactory outcomes. Of the patients with satisfactory outcomes, all ten reported no additional episodes of instability and had less apprehension on physical exam. Two of the three unsatisfactory outcomes noted recurrence of their anterior instability, which occurred after additional traumatic events.

Resch et al. [17] reported on 12 patients with irreparable subscapularis ruptures, at an average follow-up of 28 months, which were treated with a split pectoralis major subcoracoid transfer. Patients were assessed on strength, range of motion, Constant scores, and patient reported subjective assessment. On subjective assessment, nine were excellent/good, three were fair, and none were poor. Pain scores improved from 1.7 out of 15 preoperatively to 9.6 out of 15 postoperatively. Constant scores increased from 26.9 to 67.1 % of normal following surgery. No patients had recurrence of anterior instability.

Galatz et al. [13] reported on 14 patients with irreparable subscapularis tears with associated anterosuperior instability who were treated with subcoracoid pectoralis major transfers of the entire tendon. The mean follow-up was 17.5 months, and at that time point there were 11 satisfactory and 3 unsatisfactory results. Pain scores, on the visual analog scale, decreased from 6.9 to 3.2 postoperatively. ASES functional outcome scores increased from 27.2 to 47.7 following surgery. Seven patients had full containment of the humeral head; six patients had intermediate instability, defined as some instability at initiation

of elevation; and one patient with an uncontained humeral head. Of note, the patients in this study also had the following procedures: one deltoidplasty, two attempted rotator cuff repairs, two biceps tenodeses, one heterotopic ossification excision, one revision total shoulder arthroplasty, one hemiarthroplasty, three revision hemiarthroplasties, two repeat irrigation and debridements, one intercalary allograft of the proximal humerus, one Achilles tendon allograft reconstruction of the coracoacromial arch, and two patients had sutures weaved around the humeral head to augment humeral head containment. Complications included one patient with transient neuropraxia of the musculocutaneous nerve and one patient with rupture of the transferred pectoralis major tendon.

Jost et al. [15] reported on 28 patients who underwent 30 pectoralis major transfers for an irreparable subscapularis tear, with or without associated superior rotator cuff tears. The transfers were performed using the entire pectoralis major and was passed anterior to the conjoined tendon. Mean follow-up in this series was 32 months. The Constant scores improved from 47 to 70 % following surgery. Patients reported they were very satisfied in 14 shoulders, satisfied in 10 shoulders, disappointed in 3 shoulders, and dissatisfied in 3 shoulders. When the patients with associated irreparable supraspinatus tears were compared with isolated irreparable subscapularis tears, it was noted that the Constant scores were statistically significantly better, at 49 % versus 79 %, with the isolated subscapularis tears. The authors reported six postoperative complications including two ruptures of the transferred pectoralis tendon, one reruption of a repaired supraspinatus and infraspinatus, one infection, one axillary vein thrombosis, and one case of impingement between the humeral head and the coracoid process.

Warner [59] reported on ten patients with irreparable subscapularis ruptures who underwent split pectoralis major transfer, of the sternal head, anterior to the conjoined tendon. All patients reported of a stable shoulder and had improvement in pain scores, but only six of the ten reported minimal or no pain. Functional gains were less impressive with five patients reporting minimal functional improvement, three patients reported some functional improvement but noted limitations with overhead activities, and two patients noted marked improvement with the ability to return to most activities including sports such as golf and tennis. No complications were reported.

Elhassan et al. [12] reported on 30 patients who underwent supracoracoid split pectoralis major transfer for irreparable subscapularis for three distinct subsets of patients. Group I were patients with a failed procedure for anterior instability, group II were patients with anterior instability following shoulder arthroplasty, and group III were massive, irreparable tears of the anterosuperior rotator cuff. The pain scores improved in 7 of the 11 patients in groups I and III, but only 1 of the 8 patients in group II noted pain improvement. The subjective shoulder scores improved in 7 of 11 patients in group I, 1 of 8 patients in group II, and 6 of 11 patients in group III. The mean Constant scores improved from 40.9 to 60.8 in group I, 32.9 to 41.9 in group II, and 28.7 to 52.3 in group III. The authors also noted the failure rates were highest in group II and was associated with preoperative anterior subluxation of the humeral head. They concluded patients with subscapularis insufficiency following shoulder arthroplasty are at a higher risk for failure following pectoralis major transfers. No complications other than ruptures of the transferred tendon were reported.

Conclusions

Isolated tears of the subscapularis are less frequently encountered than those of the superior rotator cuff, and their clinical presentation can be notably subtle. The management of irreparable subscapularis tears can be challenging, with the current workhorse procedure being the transfer of all or a portion of the pectoralis major tendon. There are a few described techniques in the literature, with the most notable areas of distinction being the amount of the pectoralis being transferred (all or split) and the positioning of the transferred musculotendinous unit as it relates to

the coracoid process and conjoined tendon. Based on results presented in a number of small clinical series after this procedure, improvement in pain and incremental functional gains can be expected after this procedure in the majority of patients.

References

1. Codman EA. Lesions of the supraspinatus tendon and other lesions in or about the subacromial bursa. In: The shoulder. Boston: Thomas Todd Co; 1934. p. 65–7.
2. Deutsch A, Altchek DW, Veltri DM, Potter HG, Warren RF. Traumatic tears of the subscapularis tendon. Clinical diagnosis, magnetic resonance imaging findings, and operative treatment. Am J Sports Med. 1997;25:13–22.
3. Frankle MA, Cofield RH. Rotator cuff tears involving the subscapularis tendon. Techniques and results of repair. In: Proceedings of the fifth international conference on Shoulder Surgery; 12–15 Jul 1992; Paris. International Shoulder and Elbow Society; 1992. p. 52.
4. Bennett WF. Subscapularis, medial, and lateral head coracohumeral ligament insertion anatomy: arthroscopic appearance and incidence of "hidden" rotator interval lesions. Arthroscopy. 2001;17:173–80.
5. Ticker JB, Burkhart SS. Why repair the subscapularis? A logical rationale. Arthroscopy. 2011;27:1123–8.
6. Gerber C, Krushell RJ. Isolated rupture of the tendon of the subscapularis muscle. Clinical features in 16 cases. J Bone Joint Surg Br. 1991;73:389–94.
7. Warner JJ, Higgins L, Parsons 4th IM, Dowdy P. Diagnosis and treatment of anterosuperior rotator cuff tears. J Shoulder Elbow Surg. 2001;10:37–46.
8. Goutallier D, Postel JM, Bernageau J, Lavau L, Voisin MC. Fatty muscle degeneration in cuff ruptures. Pre- and post-operative evaluation by CT scan. Clin Orthop Relat Res. 1994;304:78–83.
9. Goutallier D, Postel JM, Gleyze P, Leguilloux P, Van Driessche S. Influence of cuff muscle fatty degeneration on anatomic and functional outcomes after simple suture of full-thickness tears. J Shoulder Elbow Surg. 2003;12:550–4.
10. Mellado JM, Calmet J, Olona M, Esteve C, Camins A, Perez Del Palomar L, et al. Surgically repaired massive rotator cuff tears: MRI of tendon integrity, muscle fatty degeneration, and muscle atrophy correlated with intraoperative and clinical findings. Am J Roentgenol. 2005;184:1456–63.
11. Thomazeau H, Boukobza E, Morcet N, Chaperon J, Langlais F. Prediction of rotator cuff repair results by magnetic resonance imaging. Clin Orthop Relat Res. 1997;344:275–83.
12. Elhassan B, Ozbaydar M, Massimini D, Diller D, Higgins L, Warner JJ. Transfer of pectoralis major for

the treatment of irreparable tears of subscapularis: does it work? J Bone Joint Surg Br. 2008;90:1059–65.

13. Galatz LM, Connor PM, Calfee RP, Hsu JC, Yamaguchi K. Pectoralis major transfer for anterior-superior subluxation in massive rotator cuff insufficiency. J Shoulder Elbow Surg. 2003;12:1–5.

14. Gavriilidis I, Kircher J, Magosch P, Licthenberg S, Habermeyer P. Pectoralis major transfer for the treatment of irreparable anterosuperior rotator cuff tears. Int Orthop. 2010;34:689–94.

15. Jost B, Puskas GJ, Lustenberger A, Gerber C. Outcome of pectoralis major transfer for the treatment of irreparable subscapularis tears. J Bone Joint Surg Am. 2003;85-A:1944–51.

16. Lederer S, Auffarth A, Bogner R, Tauber M, Mayer M, Karpik S, Matis N, Resch H. Magnetic resonance imaging-controlled results of the pectoralis major tendon transfer for irreparable anterosuperior rotator cuff tears performed with standard and modified fixation techniques. J Shoulder Elbow Surg. 2011;20:1155–62.

17. Resch H, Povacz P, Ritter E, Matschi W. Transfer of the pectoralis major muscle for the treatment of irreparable rupture of the subscapularis tendon. J Bone Joint Surg Am. 2000;82:372–82.

18. Wirth MA, Rockwood Jr CA. Operative treatment of irreparable rupture of the subscapularis. J Bone Joint Surg Am. 1997;79:722–73.

19. DePalma AF. Surgery of the shoulder. Philadelphia: Lippincott; 1950. p. 209–20.

20. Li XX, Schweitzer ME, Bifano JA, Lerman J, Manton GL, El-Noueam KI. MR evaluation of subscapularis tears. J Comput Assist Tomogr. 1999;23:713–7.

21. Arai R, Sugaya H, Mochizuki T, Nimura A, Moriishi J, Akita K. Subscapularis tendon tear: an anatomic and clinical investigation. Arthroscopy. 2008;24:997–1004.

22. Barth JR, Burkhart SS, De Beer JF. The bear-hug test: a new and sensitive test for diagnosing a subscapularis tear. Arthroscopy. 2006;22:1076–84.

23. Lafosse L, Jost B, Reiland Y, Audebert S, Toussaint B, Gobezie R. Structural integrity and clinical outcomes after arthroscopic repair of isolated subscapularis tears. J Bone Joint Surg Am. 2007;89:1184–93.

24. Neviaser RJ, Neviaser TJ, Neviaser JS. Concurrent rupture of the rotator cuff and anterior dislocation of the shoulder in the older patient. J Bone Joint Surg Am. 1988;70:1308–11.

25. Nove-Josserand L, Levigne C, Noel E, Walch G. Isolated lesions of the subscapularis muscle. Apropos of 21 cases. Rev Chir Orthop Reparatrice Appar Mot. 1994;80:595–601. French.

26. Walch G, Boileau P. Rotator cuff tears associated with anterior instability. In: Warner JPJ, Iannotti JP, Gerber C, editors. Complex and revision problems in shoulder surgery. Philadelphia: Lippincott-Raven; 1997. p. 65–70.

27. Garavaglia G, Ufenast H, Taverna E. The frequency of subscapularis tear in arthroscopic rotator cuff repair: a retrospective study comparing magnetic resonance

imaging and arthroscopic findings. Int J Should Surg. 2001;5:91–4.

28. Ulrich L, Fullick R, Bongiorno V, Saintmard B, Campens C, Lafosse L. Arthroscopic repair of large subscapularis tendon tears: 2- to 4-year clinical and radiographic outcomes. Arthroscopy. 2013;29:1471–8.

29. Bennett WF. Arthroscopic repair of isolated subscapularis tears: a prospective cohort with 2- to 4-year follow-up. Arthroscopy. 2003;19:131–43.

30. Toussaint B, Audebert S, Barth J, Charousset C, Godeneche A, Joudet T, Lefebvre Y, Nove-Josserand L, Petroff E, Solignac N, Hardy P, Scymanski C, Maynou C, Thelu C-E, Boileau P, Pitermann M, Graveleau N, French Arthroscopy Society (SFA). Arthroscopic repair of subscapularis tears: preliminary data from a prospective multicentre study. Orthop Traumatol Surg Res. 2012;98(8 Suppl):S193–200.

31. Gray H. The muscles and fasciae of the shoulder. In: Goss CM, editor. Gray's anatomy of the human body. 28th ed. Philadelphia: Lea and Febiger; 1968. p. 458–9.

32. Keating JF, Waterworth P, Shaw-Dunn J, Crossan J. The relative strengths of the rotator cuff muscles. A cadaver study. J Bone Joint Surg Br. 1993;75:137–40.

33. Richards DP, Burkhart SS, Tehrany AM, Wirth MA. The subscapularis footprint: an anatomic description of its insertion site. Arthroscopy. 2007;23:251–4.

34. Kato K. Innervation of the scapular muscles and its morphological significance in man. Anat Anz. 1989; 168:155–68.

35. Iannotti JP, Gabriel JP, Schneck SL, Evans BG, Misra S. The normal glenohumeral relationships. An anatomical study of one hundred and forty shoulders. J Bone Joint Surg Am. 1992;74:491–500.

36. Burkhart SS. Arthroscopic treatment of massive rotator cuff tears: clinical results and biomechanical rationale. Clin Orthop Relat Res. 1991;267:45–56.

37. Burkhart SS. Fluoroscopic comparison of kinematic patterns in massive rotator cuff tears. A suspension bridge model. Clin Orthop Relat Res. 1992;(284):144–52.

38. David G, Magarey ME, Jones MA, Dvir Z, Türker KS, Sharpe M. EMG and strength correlates of selected shoulder muscles during rotations of the glenohumeral joint. Clin Biomech (Bristol, Avon). 2000; 15:95–102.

39. Denard PJ, Lädermann A, Burkhart SS. Arthroscopic management of subscapularis tears. Sports Med Arthrosc. 2011;19:333–41.

40. Inman VT, Saunders JB, Abbott LC. Observations on the function of the shoulder joint. J Bone Joint Surg. 1944;26:1–30.

41. Thompson WO, Debski RE, Boardman 3rd ND, Taskiran E, Warner JJ, Fu FH, et al. A biomechanical analysis of rotator cuff deficiency in a cadaveric model. Am J Sports Med. 1996;24:286–92.

42. Gerber C, Hersche O, Farron A. Isolated rupture of the subscapularis tendon. Results of operative repair. J Bone Joint Surg Am. 1996;78:1015–23.

43. Hegedus EJ, Goode AP, Cook CE, Michener L, Myer CA, Myer DM, et al. Which physical examination tests provide clinicians with the most value when examining the shoulder? Update of a systematic review with meta-analysis of individual tests. Br J Sports Med. 2012;46:964–78.

44. Hertel R, Ballmer FT, Lambert SM, Gerber C. Lag signs in the diagnosis of rotator cuff rupture. J Shoulder Elbow Surg. 1996;5:307–13.

45. Pennock AT, Pennington WW, Torry MR, Decker MJ, Vaishnav SB, Provencher MT, Millett PJ, Hackett TR. The influence of arm and shoulder position on the bear-hug, belly-press, and lift-off tests: an electromyographic study. Am J Sports Med. 2011;39:2338–46.

46. Scheibel M, Magosch P, Pritsch M, Lichtenberg S, Habermeyer P. The belly-off sign: a new clinical diagnostic sign for subscapularis lesions. Arthroscopy. 2005;21:1229–35.

47. Ballmer FT, Lambert SM, Hertel R. Napoleon's sign: a test to assess subscapularis function. J Shoulder Elbow Surg. 1997;6:193.

48. Scheibel M, Tsynman A, Magosch P, Schroeder RJ, Habermeyer P. Postoperative subscapularis muscle insufficiency after primary and revision open shoulder stabilization. Am J Sports Med. 2006;34:1586–93.

49. Burkhart SS, Tehrany AM. Arthroscopic subscapularis tendon repair: technique and preliminary results. Arthroscopy. 2002;18:454–63.

50. Schwamborn T, Imhoff AB. Diagnosis and classification of rotator cuff lesions. In: Imhoff AB, Konig U, editors. Schulterinstabilitat-Rotatorenmanschette. Darmstadt: Steinkopff Verlag; 1999. p. 193–5. German.

51. Bartsch M, Greiner S, Haas NP, Scheibel M. Diagnostic values of clinical tests for subscapularis lesions. Knee Surg Sports Traumatol Arthrosc. 2010;18:1712–7.

52. Rigsby R, Sitler M, Kelly JD. Subscapularis tendon integrity: an examination of shoulder index tests. J Athl Train. 2010;45:404–6.

53. Teefey SA, Hasan SA, Middleton WD, Patel M, Wright RW, Yamaguchi K. Ultrasonography of the rotator cuff: a comparison of ultrasonographic and arthroscopic findings in one hundred consecutive cases. J Bone Joint Surg Am. 2000;82A:498–504.

54. Hodler J, Kursunoglu-Brahme S, Snyder SJ, Cervilla V, Karzel RP, Schweitzer ME, et al. Rotator cuff disease: assessment with MR arthrography versus standard MR imaging in 36 patients with arthroscopic confirmation. Radiology. 1992;182:431–6.

55. Palmer EW, Brown JH, Rosenthal DI. Rotator cuff: evaluation with fat-suppressed MR arthrography. Radiology. 1993;188:683–7.

56. Jung JY, Yoon YC, Cha DI, Yoo JC, Jung JY. The "bridging sign": a MR finding for combined full-thickness tears of the subscapularis tendon and the supraspinatus tendon. Acta Radiol. 2013;54:83–8.

57. Fuchs B, Weishaupt D, Zanetti M, Hodler J, Gerber C. Fatty degeneration of the muscles of the rotator cuff: assessment by computed tomography versus magnetic resonance imaging. J Shoulder Elbow Surg. 1999;8:599–605.

58. Omid R, Lee B. Tendon transfers for irreparable rotator cuff tears. J Am Acad Orthop Surg. 2013;21:492–501.

59. Warner JJ. Management of massive irreparable rotator cuff tears: the role of tendon transfer. Instr Course Lect. 2001;50:63–71.

60. Levy O, Mullett H, Roberts S, Copeland S. The role of anterior deltoid reeducation in patients with massive irreparable degenerative rotator cuff tears. J Shoulder Elbow Surg. 2008;17:863–70.

61. Cofield R, Parvizi J, Hoffmeyer P, Lanzer W, Ilstrup D, Rowland C. Surgical repair of chronic rotator cuff tears: a prospective long-term study. J Bone Joint Surg Am. 2001;83:71–7.

62. Gerber C, Fuchs B, Hodler J. The results of repair of massive tears of the rotator cuff. J Bone Joint Surg Am. 2000;82:505–15.

63. Keener J, Wei A, Kim H, Steger-May K, Yamaguchi K. Proximal humeral migration in shoulders with symptomatic and asymptomatic rotator cuff tears. J Bone Joint Surg Am. 2009;91:1405–13.

64. Melillo AS, Savoie 3rd FH, Field LD. Massive rotator cuff tears: debridement versus repair. Orthop Clin North Am. 1997;28:117–24.

65. Burkart S, Nottage W, Ogilvie-Harris D, Kohn H, Pachelli A. Partial repair of irreparable rotator cuff tears. Arthroscopy. 1994;10:363–70.

66. Flatow E, Connor P, Levine W. Coracoacromial arch reconstruction for anterosuperior subluxation after failed rotator cuff surgery. J Shoulder Elbow Surg. 1997;6:228.

67. Mulieri P, Dunning P, Klein S, Pupello D, Frankle M. Reverse shoulder arthroplasty for the treatment of irreparable rotator cuff tear without glenohumeral arthritis. J Bone Joint Surg Am. 2010;92:2544–56.

68. Flatow E, Bigliani LU, April EW. An anatomic study of the musculocutaneous nerve and its relationship to the coracoid. Clin Orthop Relat Res. 1989;244:166–71.

69. Klepps SJ, Goldfarb C, Flatow E, Galatz L, Yamaguchi K. Anatomic evaluation of the subcoracoid pectoralis major transfer in human cadavers. J Shoulder Elbow Surg. 2001;10:453–9.

Hemiarthroplasty

9

Seth C. Gamradt

Disclosure: The senior author (SCG) is a consultant for Biomet.

S.C. Gamradt, MD (✉)
Department of Orthopaedic Surgery,
Keck School of Medicine of University
of Southern California, 1520 San Pablo Street,
Suite 200, Los Angeles, CA 90033, USA
e-mail: Gamradt@usc.edu

Background

Prior to the advent of the reverse total shoulder arthroplasty, hemiarthroplasty was considered the prosthesis of choice when treating cuff tear arthropathy (CTA) with arthroplasty as implantation of a conventional total shoulder arthroplasty resulted in early glenoid component loosening [1]. Several authors have described the results of hemiarthroplasty in the setting of massive rotator cuff tearing and cuff tear arthropathy (CTA). Conventional thinking is that hemiarthroplasty in the setting of advanced cuff disease can provide some pain relief while improving function only marginally. Therefore, among experienced shoulder arthroplasty surgeons, the hemiarthroplasty was offered to CTA patients with a healthy dose of pessimism due to a large number of patients with persistent unfavorable pain relief and/or limited gain in function.

Over the past decade, the indications for hemiarthroplasty in the cuff-deficient shoulder have diminished even further with the advent and widespread acceptance of the reverse arthroplasty

Table 9.1 Indications for hemiarthroplasty in the cuff-deficient shoulder

Cuff tear arthropathy in the elderly, low-demand patient desiring only pain relief and a low-risk operation (Fig. 9.1)
Cuff tear arthropathy or massive rotator cuff tear with preoperative forward elevation greater than 90° (Fig. 9.2)

Table 9.2 Contraindications to hemiarthroplasty in the cuff-deficient shoulder

Pseudoparalysis or preoperative forward elevation less than 90°
Insufficient coracoacromial arch and/or previous acromioplasty
Anterosuperior escape
Infection
Deltoid dysfunction
Absent or torn subscapularis

as the preferred surgical treatment for CTA with anterosuperior escape and pseudoparalysis. This chapter examines the past and current literature in an attempt to update the current role (albeit somewhat limited) of hemiarthroplasty as treatment for the cuff-deficient shoulder (Tables 9.1 and 9.2).

Description of the Technique

The hemiarthroplasty for a cuff-deficient shoulder is technically not challenging when compared to reverse arthroplasty or conventional total shoulder arthroplasty in shoulders with an intact cuff. Goldberg and Bigliani provide an excellent description of the surgical technique [2]. A modified beach chair position is used. A mechanical arm holder is useful. A deltopectoral approach is used protecting the cephalic vein. Blunt dissection is used to expose the subacromial, subdeltoid, and subconjoined spaces. A self-retaining retractor is used to expose the subscapularis with the blades beneath the conjoined tendon and the deltoid. The biceps is tenotomized for later tenodesis if present. A subscapularis tenotomy is performed carefully tagging the tendon for later repair. The anterior humeral circumflex vessels are ligated or coagulated at the muscular portion of the inferior subscapularis.

Progressive extension and external rotation are used to dislocate the humeral head. Due to the massive tearing of the rotator cuff, exposure of the humerus is easily gained. An intramedullary guide can be used to guide a humeral cut in anatomic retroversion (about 30°). The height of the cut should aim to exit superiorly at the level of the greater tuberosity. After the humeral head cut, we mobilize any remaining supraspinatus and infraspinatus for later repair to the greater tuberosity.

Broaches are used to prepare the canal in standard fashion, and the final broach is used to trial extended coverage humeral heads that are designed to articulate with the acromion. Final tension should allow the humerus to glide about fifty percent anteriorly and posteriorly without instability. After ensuring an adequate fit of the prosthesis, definitive implants are inserted in standard fashion. Prior to placement of the definitive press-fit humeral stem, we pass heavy #5 suture through the lesser tuberosity to facilitate subscapularis repair. In addition, at this point, sutures can be passed through the greater tuberosity to aid in repairing as much rotator cuff as possible.

Currently, some modern shoulder systems allow for conversion of a hemiarthroplasty to reverse arthroplasty without removal of the stem. At present, we recommend using this type of convertible or modular stem to avoid having to extract a stem if the patient requires conversion to reverse arthroplasty at some point in the future. A partial rotator cuff repair is undertaken then with the sutures passed through the greater tuberosity. The subscapularis is then closed through drill holes in the lesser tuberosity or by using a tendon-to-tendon stitch (see Pearls and Pitfalls and Table 9.3).

Outcomes

Several classic articles must be mentioned when discussing the outcomes of hemiarthroplasty in the cuff-deficient shoulder. Williams et al. reviewed the results of 21 hemiarthroplasties performed in the setting of rotator cuff deficiency [3]. Using Neer's grading scale for shoulder arthro-

Table 9.3 Rehabilitation

Healing phase: (week 0–6) in a sling to protect the subscapularis repair and cuff repair (if performed)
Allow immediate passive forward elevation, pendulums, isometric deltoid exercises
Protect external rotation to neutral
Motion phase (week 6–12)
Allow active, active-assisted, and gentle passive ROM in all planes
Gentle strengthening at waist level
Strength phase (week 12 and beyond)
Progressive resistance exercises
Strength goals are limited in this population, and we proceed with anterior deltoid strengthening with the Levy protocol for massive rotator cuff tearing

plasty, there were no excellent results, 14 satisfactory results, and 7 unsatisfactory results. Active forward flexion improved from 70° preoperatively to 120° postoperatively. Similarly, Zuckerman et al. reviewed the results of 15 hemiarthroplasty for rotator cuff arthropathy. At a mean follow-up of 28.2 months, patients gained a modest improvement in forward elevation from 69° to 86°; 14 of 15 patients had significant pain relief [4].

Sanchez Sotelo and the group from the Mayo Clinic evaluated the results of hemiarthroplasty for glenohumeral arthritis associated with rotator cuff deficiency. At an average of 5-year follow-up, 33 shoulders showed an average gain of forward elevation to 91° from 72°. There were 11 unsuccessful results [5].

Taken together, these historical results of hemiarthroplasty in the setting of CTA show that while hemiarthroplasty clearly provides pain relief, functional improvement is less predictable with many patients improving their range of motion only marginally; also, there is a subset of patients (up to a third) who remain dissatisfied with the operation.

More recent results echo these older results. Vistosky et al. retrospectively reviewed the results of 60 patients that received hemiarthroplasty with an extended coverage humeral head for treatment of rotator cuff tear arthropathy [6]. These authors showed the most dramatic improvement in range of motion across the previous studies mentioned with forward elevation improving from 56° to

116° in patients with 2-year follow-up. Importantly, the visual analog pain scale improved from 9.3 preoperatively to 1.9 postoperatively. To date, there have been no comparative trials evaluating the effectiveness of the extended coverage humeral head (CTA head) in comparison to a conventional hemiarthroplasty.

Goldberg et al. retrospectively evaluated the results of hemiarthroplasty in 31 patients with 34 cuff-deficient shoulders [7]. Average forward elevation improved from 78° to 111° postoperatively. The most important finding of this study was that patients that had preoperative forward elevation of greater than 90° had higher final ASES scores (both total and functional) and better pain relief when compared to patients with worse preoperative motion. In addition to hemiarthroplasty in the study, all patients in these series had an attempt at partial or complete cuff repair with a trend toward improved results in those patients in which a repair was possible.

While it is clear that hemiarthroplasty can provide some benefit to certain patients, there are data that show that among indications for hemiarthroplasty, CTA is one of the least favorable. Hettrich et al. retrospectively studied 71 hemiarthroplasties in an attempt to identify preoperative factors associated with a good functional result [8]. An intact rotator cuff was a predictor for improved function postoperatively and a diagnosis of cuff tear arthropathy (along with capsulorrhaphy arthropathy and rheumatoid arthritis) showed the least functional shoulder improvement.

In a large study (272 shoulders) evaluating the outcomes and long-term survival analysis according to etiology, Gadea et al. showed that the rotator cuff arthropathy as a preoperative diagnosis resulted in a 10-year survival rate of 81.5 % but a low Constant-Murley score (46.2) [9]. The authors concluded that the best indications for hemiarthroplasty in their group of patients was avascular necrosis and that the worst indications were cuff tear arthropathy and fracture sequelae.

Although there are few prospectively collected comparative data regarding CTA for hemiarthroplasty, these two aforementioned studies reveal that the results of hemiarthroplasty for

CTA are likely to inferior to the results of hemiarthroplasty for other indications in the cuff-intact shoulder such as avascular necrosis. Due to the relatively poor results with hemiarthroplasty in CTA, shoulder arthroplasty surgeons have turned increasingly to the reverse arthroplasty in the cuff-deficient shoulder [10]. However, since the advent of the reverse replacement, there have been very few studies that actually directly compare the results of reverse arthroplasty with conventional arthroplasty.

Young et al. published an important matched pair analysis of hemiarthroplasty and reverse arthroplasty in cuff tear arthropathy from the New Zealand joint replacement registry [11]. These authors compared prospectively collected data from 102 matched pairs of shoulder replacements. Patients had an average age of 71.6 years in the hemiarthroplasty group and 72.6 years in the reverse arthroplasty group. The main finding of the study was improved Oxford Shoulder Scores (mean 37.5 vs 31.1) at 6 months. In addition, six patients in the hemiarthroplasty group were revised for ongoing pain to reverse shoulder arthroplasty during the study period. The main criticism of the study is that only a limited number of patients had completed 5-year outcome scores (18 in the hemi group and 14 in the RSA group), but the difference in functional result appeared to be maintained in those patients (Figs. 9.1 and 9.2).

Leung et al. performed a retrospective case control series evaluating the functional outcomes of hemiarthroplasty versus reverse arthroplasty in the treatment of cuff tear arthropathy [12]. These authors concluded that the reverse arthroplasty group (36 patients) had better functional outcome scores and improved forward elevation in comparison to hemiarthroplasty (20 shoulders) at a minimum of 2-year follow-up. Complication rate in both groups was 25 %. An interesting finding was a significant improvement in external rotation between year 1 and year 2 for the reverse arthroplasty group. These two short-term studies, albeit not with level one evidence, show that reverse replacement results in improved shoulder function when compared to hemiarthroplasty in the setting of cuff tear arthropathy. In addition,

in a Markov decision model study, reverse arthroplasty was a cost-effective surgical strategy when compared with hemiarthroplasty [13].

Conclusions

Arthroplasty for the rotator cuff-deficient shoulder has historically been a difficult challenge facing surgeons. Most studies regarding hemiarthroplasty in the cuff-deficient shoulder are retrospective with limited follow-up. Very little comparative data are available, and there are no level-1 studies to guide indications to date. Despite the lack of high-level evidence, several institutions' retrospective case series are very similar, allowing the surgeon to draw several conclusions. These conclusions are listed below:

1. Hemiarthroplasty in the setting of massive cuff tear or early CTA will result, on average, in a modest gain of forward elevation and good but not excellent pain relief.
2. Preoperative range of motion greater than 90° is an important predictor for success of the operation with regard to both patient satisfaction and postoperative function.
3. Poor results can be expected with hemiarthroplasty in those patients with anterosuperior escape and/or pseudoparalysis.
4. Hemiarthroplasty for CTA on average results in poorer outcomes when compared to other indications such as avascular necrosis.
5. Although level one evidence is lacking, there are comparative data that show that hemiarthroplasty results in slightly inferior functional results when compared to reverse arthroplasty in the setting of cuff tear arthropathy.
6. A certain subset of patients (up to a third) are unhappy with the results of hemiarthroplasty in CTA and a significant number of patients can end up needing conversion to reverse arthroplasty.
7. Several prominent authors conclude that the best indication for hemiarthroplasty in CTA are in a younger patient (<65) with preoperative range of motion greater than 90°. The ideal

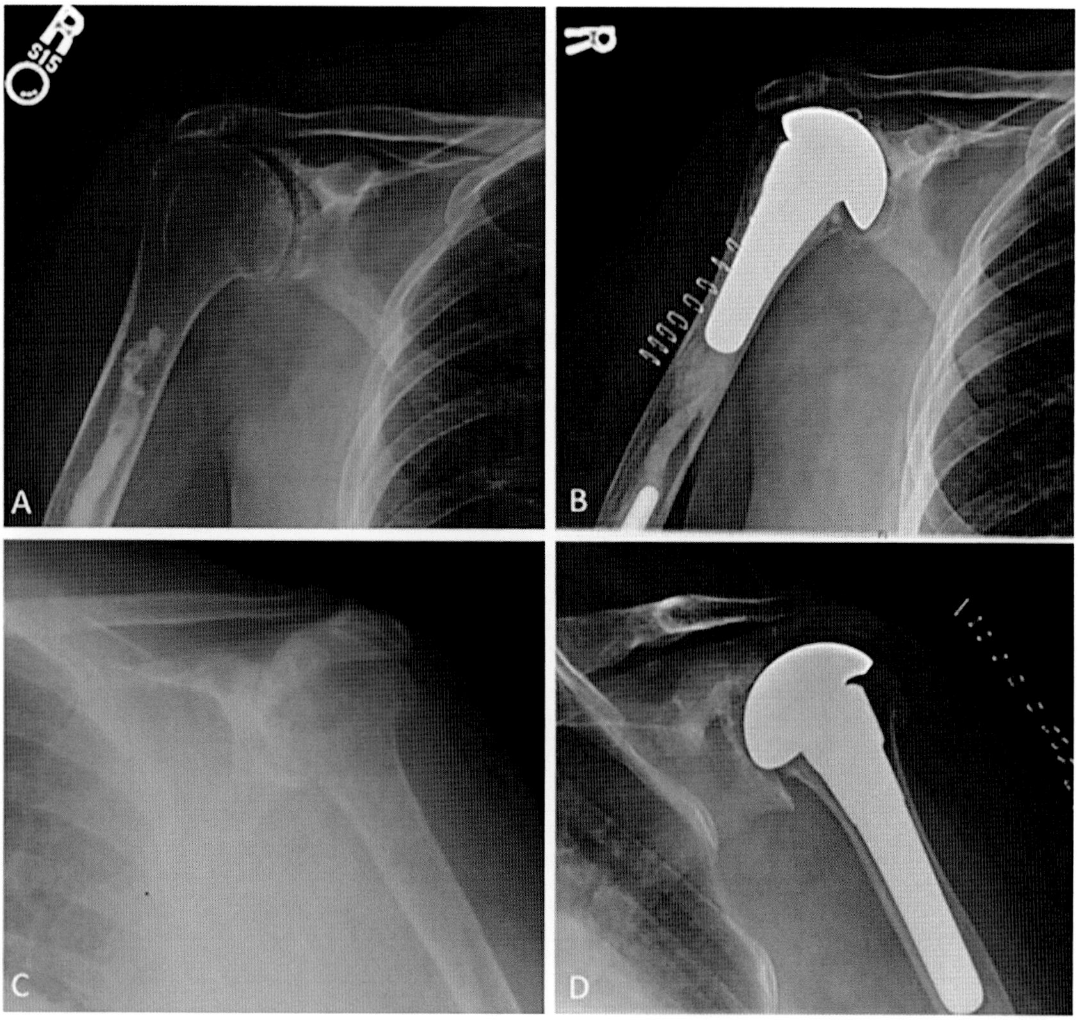

Fig. 9.1 A 75-year-old obese, low-demand woman with obesity and severe osteoporosis underwent staged bilateral hemiarthroplasty using extended articular surface heads. The patient had grade 4 atrophy of supraspinatus and infraspinatus but an intact subscapularis and an intact coracoacromial arch. Forward elevation increased from 60° bilaterally to 80° bilaterally and pain relief was excellent (**a**, **c**: preoperative radiographs, **b**, **d**: postoperative radiographs)

candidate would also have an intact subscapularis, no pseudoparalysis, and an intact coracoacromial arch [10, 14–16].

Clearly the advent of the reverse replacement has dramatically reduced the indications for hemiarthroplasty in the cuff-deficient shoulder and in rotator cuff arthropathy. Non-randomized but comparative literature have shown that outcome scores are improved with respect to patient function and forward elevation when reverse arthroplasty is compared with conventional hemiarthroplasty. The benefits of a hemiarthroplasty in comparison to reverse replacement include a shorter, technically easier surgery with low chance of complication. However, the low chance of surgical complication may be outweighed by the high chance of continued symptoms, patient dissatisfaction, and eventual need to convert to reverse arthroplasty in the future. The main unknown in the literature regarding this topic is that there are very little prospectively collected long-term data evaluating either

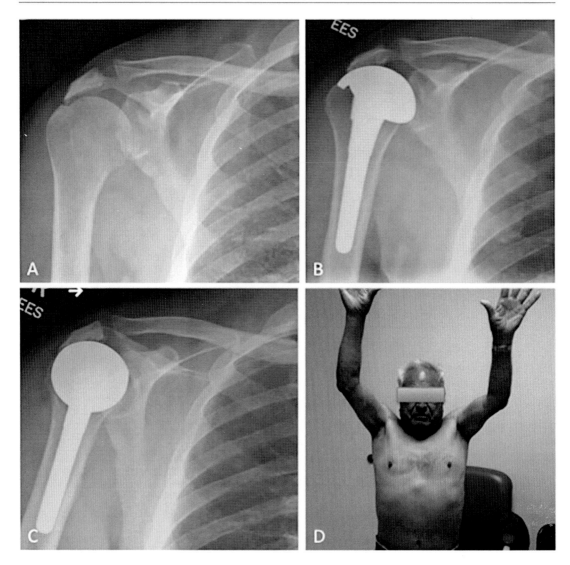

Fig. 9.2 A 65-year-old man with cuff tear arthropathy and active forward elevation preoperatively of 100° underwent staged bilateral hemiarthroplasty using extended articular surface heads. The patient had under- gone previous shoulder arthroscopy but had an intact cor- acoacromial arch (**a**: preoperative radiograph, **b**, **c**: postoperative radiographs). A modest gain in forward elevation was observed (**d**) and pain relief was excellent

hemiarthroplasty or reverse arthroplasty for CTA. There is some evidence that in 6–10-year follow-up of reverse arthroplasty, pain can return and function can deteriorate [17]. The unknown long-term durability of the reverse prosthesis may play a role in choice of prosthesis for CTA in the future, especially in younger patients.

In summary, hemiarthroplasty can be considered in the younger patient with preoperative with active forward elevation past 90°, an intact coracoacromial arch, no anterosuperior escape or high-riding humeral head, and perhaps a rotator cuff that may be amenable to a partial or complete repair. Modest gains in forward elevation and improved pain can be expected. Hemiarthroplasty should be avoided in patients with anterosuperior escape and pseudoparalysis as reverse arthroplasty has supplanted hemiarthroplasty as the surgical treatment of choice in advanced CTA. Most importantly, if a hemiarthroplasty is going to be used in CTA, it is critical to have a preoperative discussion outlining the limitations of the hemiarthroplasty and the potential for limited improvement in function and pain that could result in reverse arthroplasty conversion at some point in the future.

References

1. Franklin JL, Barrett WP, Jackins SE, Matsen 3rd FA. Glenoid loosening in total shoulder arthroplasty. Association with rotator cuff. J Arthroplasty. 1988; 3(1):39–46.
2. Goldberg SS, Bigliani LU. Hemiarthroplasty for the rotator cuff-deficient shoulder. Surgical technique. J Bone Joint Surg Am. 2009;91(Suppl 2 Pt 1):22–9.
3. Williams Jr GR, Rockwood Jr CA. Hemiarthroplasty in rotator cuff-deficient shoulders. J Shoulder Elbow Surg. 1996;5(5):362–7.
4. Zuckerman JD, Scott AJ, Gallagher MA. Hemiarthroplasty for cuff tear arthropathy. J Shoulder Elbow Surg. 2000;9(3):169–72.
5. Sanchez-Sotelo J, Cofield RH, Rowland CM. Shoulder hemiarthroplasty for glenohumeral arthritis associated with severe rotator cuff deficiency. J Bone Joint Surg Am. 2001;83-a(12):1814–22.
6. Visotsky JL, Basamania C, Seebauer L, Rockwood CA, Jensen KL. Cuff tear arthropathy: pathogenesis, classification, and algorithm for treatment. J Bone Joint Surg. 2004;86 Suppl 2:35–40.
7. Goldberg SS, Bell JE, Kim HJ, Bak SF, Levine WN, Bigliani LU. Hemiarthroplasty for the rotator cuff-deficient shoulder. J Bone Joint Surg Am. 2008; 90(3):554–9.
8. Hettrich CM, Weldon 3rd E, Boorman RS, Parsons 4th IM, Matsen 3rd FA. Preoperative factors associated with improvements in shoulder function after. J Bone Joint Surg Am. 2004;86-a(7):1446–51.
9. Gadea F, Alami G, Pape G, Boileau P, Favard L. Shoulder hemiarthroplasty: outcomes and long-term survival analysis according to etiology. Orthop Traumatol Surg Res. 2012;98(6):659–65.
10. Feeley BT, Gallo RA, Craig EV. Cuff tear arthropathy: current trends in diagnosis and surgical management. J Shoulder Elbow Surg. 2009;18(3):484–94.
11. Young SW, Zhu M, Walker CG, Poon PC. Comparison of functional outcomes of reverse shoulder arthroplasty with those of hemiarthroplasty in the treatment of cuff-tear arthropathy: a matched-pair analysis. J Bone Joint Surg Am. 2013;95(10):910–5.
12. Leung B, Horodyski M, Struk AM, Wright TW. Functional outcome of hemiarthroplasty compared with reverse total shoulder. J Shoulder Elbow Surg. 2012;21(3):319–23.
13. Coe MP, Greiwe RM, Joshi R, Snyder BM, Simpson L, Tosteson AN, et al. The cost-effectiveness of reverse total shoulder arthroplasty compared with hemiarthroplasty for rotator cuff tear arthropathy. J Shoulder Elbow Surg. 2012;21(10):1278–88.
14. Khair MM, Gulotta LV. Treatment of irreparable rotator cuff tears. Curr Rev Musculoskelet Med. 2011;4(4):208–13.
15. Macaulay AA, Greiwe RM, Bigliani LU. Rotator cuff deficient arthritis of the glenohumeral joint. Clin Orthop Surg. 2010;2(4):196–202.
16. Wiater JM, Fabing MH. Shoulder arthroplasty: prosthetic options and indications. J Am Acad Orthop Surg. 2009;17(7):415–25.
17. Guery J, Favard L, Sirveaux F, Oudet D, Mole D, Walch G. Reverse total shoulder arthroplasty. Survivorship analysis of eighty replacements. J Bone Joint Surg Am. 2006;88(8):1742–7.

Reverse Total Shoulder Arthroplasty

10

Phillip N. Williams and Edward V. Craig

Pearls and Pitfalls

Pearls

- Clarify preoperatively whether the issue is pain, lack of elevation, or lack of strength and whether severe external rotation weakness (hornblower's sign) might warrant addition of a latissimus transfer.
- Obtain a CT scan with or without three-dimensional reconstruction to evaluate available glenoid bone and pattern of bone loss. Occasionally a custom glenoid baseplate or bone grafting may be needed if there is no adequate bone for a standard glenosphere.
- At the time of surgery, especially in the presence of poor cuff tissue, residual cuff can be excised, but try to save the teres minor for some external rotation. Once the subscapularis is divided, it may or may not be able to be repaired.
- Particularly if the humeral head has been high-riding for a long period of time, a more generous humeral head osteotomy may need to be taken to seat the implant appropriately under glenosphere.
- The baseplate should have some inferior tilt and, if possible, be inferiorly seated to minimize potential for notching.
- Ideally, at least 80 % of the base plate should be seated and secured to satisfactory glenoid bone.
- Once the humeral bearing surface is inserted, proper tension in the system may be difficult to define—but, in general, should be secure when reduced and be stable throughout the full range of motion. The senior author uses "a little hard to reduce, a little hard to dislocate" as a guide or "Three Bears" analogy—not too loose, not too tight, but just right.
- It does not seem critical to repair the subscapularis, and repair may not be possible if there is poor tissue quality.
- Immobilize in a sling postoperatively—but the period of immobilization is shorter than in an anatomic total shoulder

P.N. Williams, MD
Department of Orthopaedic Surgery,
Hospital for Special Surgery, 535 E 70th Street,
New York, NY 10021, USA
e-mail: WilliamsP@hss.edu

E.V. Craig, MD, MPH (✉)
Professor of Clinical Surgery, Weill Cornell
Medical School, New York, NY, USA

Attending Surgeon, Hospital for Special Surgery, 535
E 70th Street, New York, NY 10021, USA
e-mail: CraigE@hss.edu

L.V. Gulotta and E.V. Craig (eds.), *Massive Rotator Cuff Tears: Diagnosis and Management*,
DOI 10.1007/978-1-4899-7494-5_10, © Springer Science+Business Media New York 2015

replacement in which subscapularis healing is so critical.

- If performed for fracture, repair the tuberosities for optimal functional result.

Pitfalls

- Protect the axillary nerve—loss of deltoid function is a major problem if RTSA is being performed.
- Confirm baseplate security and taper of parts are engaged fully.
- When the shoulder is reduced, make certain the arm can be brought to the side and there is no inferior impingement of the humerus on the inferior glenoid—inferior impingement can lead to prosthetic instability and scapula notching.

Rehabilitation

- Formal rehabilitation is rarely necessary after RTSA because there is frequently little cuff tissue needing postoperative protection. Postoperatively, the shoulder is immobilized in a simple sling to hold the arm in internal rotation for a few weeks. Passive range of motion is begun immediately. Afterward, the patient can remove the sling for hygiene and use the hand for simple activities of daily living. Sling use is gradually weaned after a month and activity as tolerated is permitted.

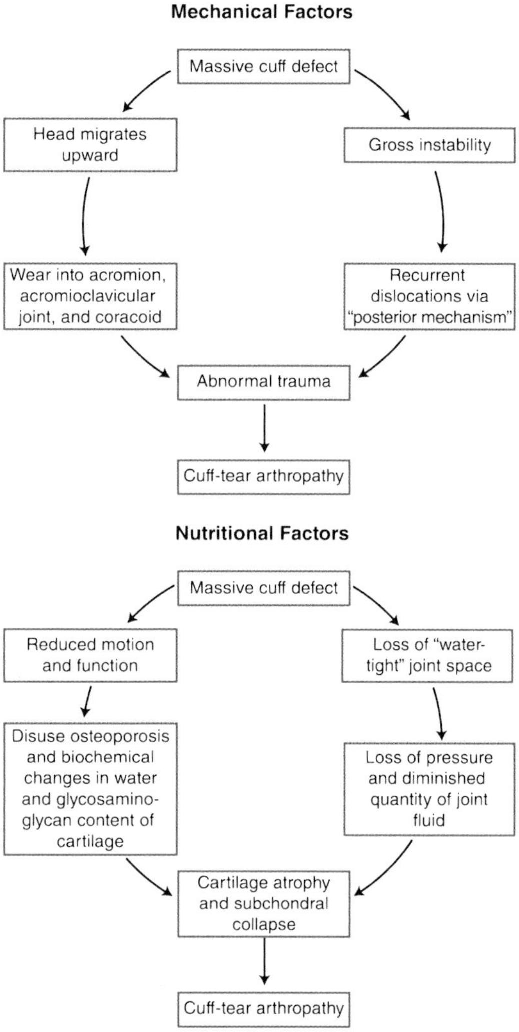

Mechanical Factors

Massive cuff defect → Head migrates upward → Wear into acromion, acromioclavicular joint, and coracoid → Abnormal trauma

Massive cuff defect → Gross instability → Recurrent dislocations via "posterior mechanism" → Abnormal trauma

Abnormal trauma → Cuff-tear arthropathy

Nutritional Factors

Massive cuff defect → Reduced motion and function → Disuse osteoporosis and biochemical changes in water and glycosaminoglycan content of cartilage → Cartilage atrophy and subchondral collapse

Massive cuff defect → Loss of "watertight" joint space → Loss of pressure and diminished quantity of joint fluid → Cartilage atrophy and subchondral collapse

Cartilage atrophy and subchondral collapse → Cuff-tear arthropathy

Fig. 10.1 Both mechanical factors (*top*) and nutritional factors (*bottom*) contribute to joint destruction in rotator cuff tear arthropathy (Modified from Neer et al. [7])

Background

The first introduction of reverse total shoulder arthroplasty (RTSA) in the 1970s was met with little clinical success. It had a constrained design and lateralized glenohumeral center of rotation that led to excessive shear forces and failure of the glenoid component [1, 2]. In the subsequent years, implant design modifications focused on a larger radius of curvature of the glenoid component and movement of the center of shoulder rotation medially and distally to decrease shear forces at the glenoid bone interface and to create a more stable and efficient deltoid fulcrum [3, 4]. Paul Grammont and colleagues modernized the reverse shoulder arthroplasty implant in 1987 to treat "cuff tear arthropathy," a clinical entity first labeled by Neer et al. [5].

Cuff tear arthropathy is shoulder arthritis in the setting of a massive, irreparable rotator cuff tear. The authors of the original Neer paper that first described the process theorized that both mechanical and nutritional factors might play a role in its development [6, 7] (Fig. 10.1).

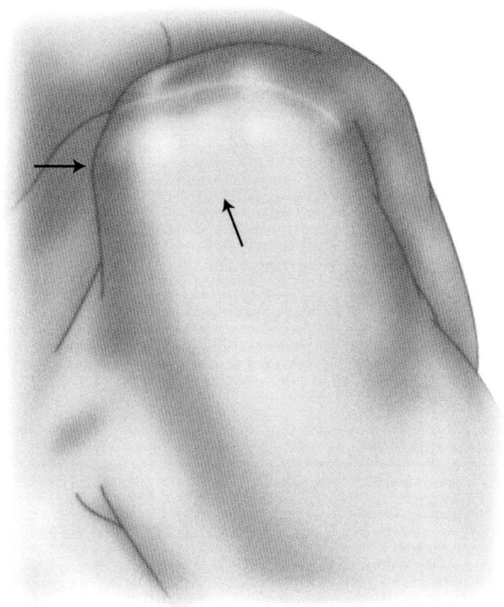

Fig. 10.2 Clinical picture of the left shoulder in a patient with rotator cuff tear arthropathy, demonstrating anterior (*left arrow*) and superior (*right arrow*) escape of the humeral head resulting from loss of the subscapularis with a grossly deficient rotator cuff (Modified from Nam et al. [8])

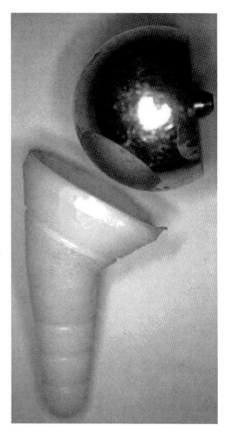

Fig. 10.3 Grammont's original reverse total shoulder arthroplasty (Reproduced with permission from Boileau et al. [12])

Mechanical factors arise from disruption of the force coupling effect, as attempts at elevation or rotation of the humerus cause instability. A deficient cuff may also allow excessive upward migration of the humeral head, resulting in abnormal pressure and degenerative changes in the acromion, acromioclavicular joint, and coracoid. In severe cases, loss of the subscapularis muscle and a grossly deficient rotator cuff lead to anterior and superior escape of the humeral head [8] (Fig. 10.2). Moreover, with attempted shoulder abduction and loss of the inferior and compressive action of the rotator cuff, the unopposed contraction of the deltoid creates a force vector that displaces the humeral head superiorly, leading to pseudoparalysis of shoulder elevation (defined as "an inability to actively elevate the arm in the presence of free passive range of motion, and in the absence of a neurologic lesion") [4]. At about the same time cuff tear arthropathy was described, the rheumatology literature reported an entity named "Milwaukee Shoulder", which was essentially the same process, and theorized that crystalline deposits had a destructive effect on both joint and soft tissue [6].

Cuff tear arthropathy treatment has ranged from nonoperative management, glenohumeral arthrodesis, resection arthroplasty, and constrained or conventional total shoulder arthroplasty to hemiarthroplasty alone [9–11]. However, these interventions resulted in poor functional outcomes and high long-term complication rates [8]. Eventually, RTSA received renewed interest once improved implant designs were able to provide glenohumeral stability and optimize shoulder biomechanics. Paul Grammont is credited with describing the modern reverse total shoulder prosthesis [12] (Fig. 10.3). Earlier reverse ball-and-socket designs included a small glenoid component and a lateralized center of rotation within the prosthesis, instead of within

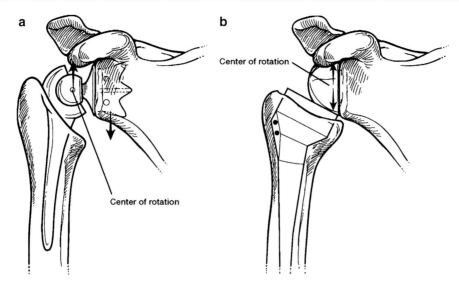

Fig. 10.4 (**a**, **b**) Diagrams demonstrating an earlier reverse total shoulder prosthesis design, with a small glenosphere component and a lateralized center of rotation (**a**), versus the modern design, with a large glenosphere, a

nonanatomic valgus angle of the humeral implant, and medial and distal positioning of the center of rotation (**b**) (Reproduced with permission from Gartsman and Edwards [13])

the glenoid. As a consequence, these designs increased stresses at the glenosphere-bone interface and led to early component failure [13] (Fig. 10.4a). The modern RTSA employs the following concepts: (1) a large glenoid component with no neck to facilitate medialization of the center of rotation and reduced torque; (2) a humeral implant with a nonanatomic valgus angle, which moves the center of joint rotation distally, thereby maximizing the length and tension of the deltoid to make it a more efficient humerus abductor, as well as increasing stability; and (3) a greater impingement-free shoulder range of motion [12, 13] (Figs. 10.4b and 10.5).

Indications

When the RTSA received US Food and Drug Administration approval in 2003, it was initially recommended only for those patients with the combination of disabling glenohumeral arthritis and cuff insufficiency. However, clinical success in restoration of stability, balance, and function has given rise to expanded indications such as the cuff deficient shoulder without arthritis. While the indications continue to evolve, concerns exist

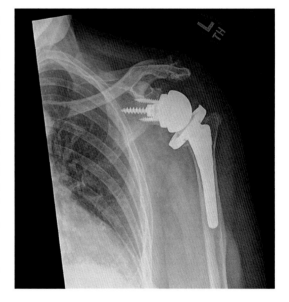

Fig. 10.5 AP radiograph of a modern reverse total shoulder arthroplasty

over its complication rate, longevity, and paucity of long-term functional outcome data [2]. Despite these concerns, the RTSA is now an important surgical option in the treatment of a variety conditions including: (1) cuff tear arthropathy, (2) irreparable cuff tears without arthritis and

Table 10.1 Indications

Cuff tear arthropathy
Pseudoparalysis
Failed cuff surgery
Anterior-superior escape
Tuberosity malunion
Acute shoulder fracture in elderly

clinical "pseudoparalysis," (3) instability directly attributable to cuff insufficiency (anterior-superior escape), (4) the "cuff insufficiency equivalent"—nonunion or malunion of the tuberosity following trauma or prior arthroplasty, (5) acute shoulder fractures in the elderly patient in which the greater tuberosity has poor potential for healing and poor bone for primary fixation, and (6) revision arthroplasty surgery. Some have recently begun to suggest its use in osteoarthritis with posterior subluxation and glenoid bone loss, a condition which has been associated on occasion with troubling posterior instability in anatomic unconstrained arthroplasty, though its use in this capacity is controversial (Table 10.1).

Cuff tear arthropathy is the single most common indication for RTSA [14]. Total shoulder replacement in the absence of a functioning rotator cuff is unpredictable in restoration of a balanced, centered shoulder, and glenoid longevity can be compromised because of the inability of the cuff to center the humeral head (rocking horse glenoid). Hemiarthroplasty with or without soft tissue interposition has had mixed results, does little to re-center the head, with few reports of improvement in active motion and functional scores [10, 15–20]. Its clinical symptoms include severe shoulder pain, shoulder or arm weakness, and progressive disability [7, 21, 22]. On exam, patients may have glenohumeral or acromiohumeral crepitus with stiffness. Rotator cuff testing will reveal specific deficiencies of the posterosuperior rotator cuff, anterosuperior, or both. Additionally, the long head of the biceps is often diseased or ruptured [7, 13, 23]. Plain radiography displays loss of glenohumeral joint space with or without humeral head osteophytes. Anterosuperior cuff failure can be appreciated on the axillary radiograph as static anterior subluxation (Fig. 10.6). If the posterosuperior

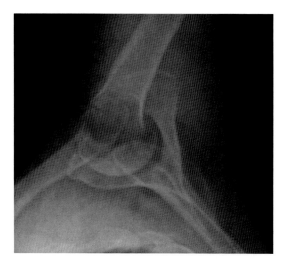

Fig. 10.6 Compromise of the anterosuperior rotator cuff results in static anterior subluxation (anterior escape) that is apparent on the axillary radiograph (Reproduced with permission from Gartsman and Edwards [13], pp 219–221)

cuff is involved, superior subluxation may be seen (Fig. 10.7). A number of studies have shown that the reverse shoulder arthroplasty can predictably restore function including overhead elevation, improve pain (as reflected in Constant score), and increase external rotation, particularly if there is a functioning teres minor [3, 24–26]. Additionally, some studies have suggested that external rotation may be reestablished with incorporation of a latissimus transfer to the reverse shoulder prosthesis [27–29].

Patients may present with massive irreparable cuff tears without glenohumeral arthritis. Despite their cuff dysfunction, some are able to compensate and maintain surprisingly good function. Thus, in the absence of arthritis, particularly if pseudoparalysis is not present, it is reasonable to attempt to build muscle through rehabilitation, allowing potential recruitment of accessory muscles. In the presence of a massive cuff tear, poor function, and pain, options other than a reverse prosthesis may include partial or complete repair, arthroscopic debridement, and biceps tenotomy. However, patients may present with pseudoparalysis: full passive forward elevation but a loss of active elevation as a result of the inability of the rotator cuff to provide a fulcrum for the deltoid during elevation.

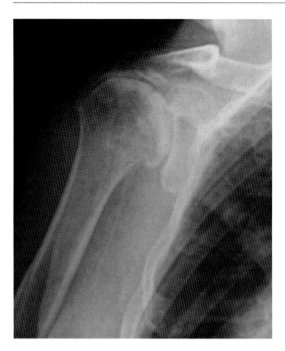

Fig. 10.7 Compromise of the posterosuperior rotator cuff results in static superior subluxation that is apparent on the anteroposterior radiograph (Reproduced with permission from Gartsman and Edwards [17], pp 219–221)

Table 10.2 Contraindications

Infection
Nonfunctioning deltoid
Insufficient glenoid bone stock/bone quality
Arthritis with a small cuff tear (relative contraindication)
Isolated external rotation pseudoparalysis (relative contraindication)

Contraindications

Infection, a nonfunctioning deltoid, and insufficient glenoid bone stock and glenoid bone quality are absolute contraindications for a RTSA. However, loss of anterior deltoid alone is not a contraindication if the middle and posterior deltoid are working effectively [30] (Table 10.2).

Arthritis and a small cuff tear with a well-centered head is a relative contraindication. In this situation a traditional anatomic arthroplasty with a cuff repair is a better alternative. Patients with massive cuff tears without arthritis and nearly full active elevation usually have a balanced shoulder with stability provided by the deltoid and residual cuff are not ideal candidates for RTSA.

RTSA cannot treat isolated external rotation deficits. The loss of active external rotation can be severely disabling and is caused from posterior extension of the rotator cuff tear to the teres minor, whereas isolated infraspinatus rupture is generally well-tolerated [31–33]. RTSA does not restore active external rotation when the posterior rotator cuff muscles are absent or deficient. Inferior outcomes have resulted from RTSA in the presence of a nonfunctioning teres minor [3, 12, 34]. Patients who regain active elevation from a RTSA but have an atrophied or absent teres minor may complain of the inability to spatially position their arm due to the tendency of their forearm to swing toward the trunk upon attempted elevation, abduction, or trying to lift an object [29]; this has clinically been termed a "hornblower's sign. A combined RTSA and latissimus dorsi and teres major transfer can restore both active elevation and external rotation in this subgroup of patients with cuff deficiency and absent or atrophied infraspinatus and teres minor [29] (Fig. 10.8).

Techniques

RTSA can be performed via a deltopectoral or a superolateral approach. There are distinct advantages and disadvantages of each approach. The argument for superolateral is that it may better ensure and provide better postoperative stability and may more effectively prevent fractures of the scapular spine and acromion [35]. A deltopectoral approach provides better preservation of active external rotation, better glenoid positioning, and easier access to the inferior glenoid, is more extensile, and may be associated with fewer incidents of inferior notching. Additionally, most surgeons are more familiar with this approach. Ultimately, the selection of approach should be based on surgeon experience and patient-specific needs. Proper implantation of a RTSA is technically demanding and should therefore be utilized

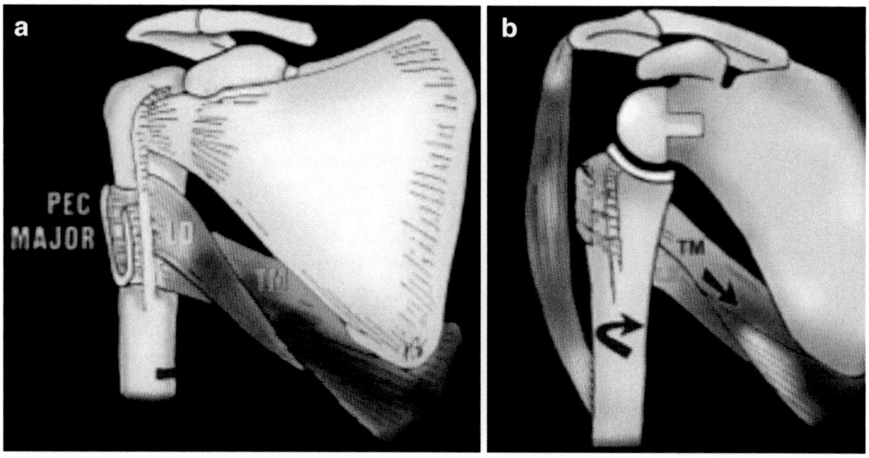

Fig. 10.8 (**a, b**) Principles of the surgical procedure are shown. The reverse prosthesis restores active elevation and the latissimus dorsi and teres major (LD/TM) transfer improves active external rotation. The two tendons that are located at the medial border of the humerus are harvested after partial section of the pectoralis major tendon (**a**). Because of the lowered, medialized position of the humerus in front of the glenosphere, the course of the rerouted tendons is short and horizontal, facilitating reattachment to the posterior aspect of the humerus (**b**) (Reproduced with permission from Boileau et al. [29])

only by experienced shoulder surgeons to minimize complications [2].

The deltopectoral approach is performed in many institutions, and it is our current preference. The key aspects will be emphasized here. The approach gives excellent humeral shaft and glenoid exposure while allowing identification and protection of the axillary nerve. The subscapularis is transected through the tendinous portion, approximately 1.5 cm medial to the insertion, in line with the anatomic neck of the humerus. It is tagged, and after prosthesis implantation, repaired with the goal of both improving humeral internal rotation and creating an anterior soft tissue restraint against instability. However, if the subscapularis is diminutive or if it cannot be repaired in a tension-free fashion with arm in 30° of external rotation, then it is not repaired. A recent retrospective case-control study found subscapularis repair conferred no appreciable effect on complication rate, dislocation events, or range of motion gains and pain relief [36]. A generous capsular release is performed along the inferior neck of the humeral head, back to the insertion of the teres minor. This will help mobilize the humerus so that better glenoid visualization can be achieved.

The specifics of humeral and glenoid preparation depend on the implant used. What follows is a general guideline for proper placement of the prosthesis. To prepare the humerus, the humeral head is typically osteotomized in anywhere between 0° and 30° of retroversion. Cutting the humerus in more retroversion is gaining favor because it may improve postoperative external rotation [37]. The long head of the biceps is tenotomized. The humerus is then reamed and broached similarly to the methods used in conventional total shoulder arthroplasty. Conveniently, many prosthesis systems are platform systems; that is, they allow the same humeral stem to be used for a hemiarthroplasty, conventional total shoulder arthroplasty, or RTSA. Such versatility affords many intraoperative options to be applied as conditions warrant and permit conversion from an anatomic arthroplasty to a reverse without the need for stem extraction (Fig. 10.9).

Once the glenoid is well-exposed, the labrum is excised and the capsule is released circumferentially. Meticulous preoperative planning with careful attention to glenoid bone stock and version is a prerequisite for proper glenoid preparation. Accurate central guidewire placement is dictated by availability of the best bone stock for

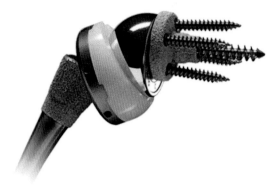

Fig. 10.9 Biomet Comprehensive® reverse shoulder system

baseplate screw fixation and placement of the baseplate as inferiorly as possible, with an inferior tilt, since this positioning has been shown to decrease the rate of implant loosening and scapular notching [32, 38, 39]. The method of baseplate fixation is system specific. An appropriate-size glenosphere is then mounted on the baseplate. Larger glenospheres may be associated with less pain and better strength [35, 40]

Once the final prosthesis is implanted and a stable range of motion is demonstrated, the subscapularis tendon is repaired and one or two suction drains are inserted. A sling is used postoperatively and the patient is allowed to use the arm for light activities of daily living such as brushing teeth and eating. Sling use is discontinued at 3 weeks in shoulders in which the subscapularis is not repaired and at 6 weeks in shoulders in which it is repaired (see Pearls and Pitfalls).

Outcomes

Results of RTSA correlate with the original indication for surgery, and functional outcome and complication rates are distinctly different in primary versus revision cases [14, 24, 25, 40]. In cuff tear arthropathy, a number of studies have shown that RTSA can predictably restore function including overhead elevation, improve pain (as reflected in Constant score), and increase external rotation, particularly if there is a functioning

teres minor [3, 24–26]. Additionally, some studies have suggested that external rotation may be reestablished with incorporation of a latissimus transfer to the reverse shoulder prosthesis when the posterior cuff and teres minor are absent or deficient [28, 29, 41]. A recent comparison of RTSA and hemiarthroplasty for the treatment of cuff tear arthropathy found superior functional outcomes for RTSA patients [42].In a large multicenter study, the Constant score increased from 24 points preoperatively to 62 points postoperatively, pain scores increased from 3.7 to 12.6 point (where 15 points represents absence of pain), and elevation increased from 71° to 130° [35]. Normalized postoperative Constant scores reflect improvement generally within the same range. Sersohn et al. [43] reported a mean of 54.3, which was similar to Ek et al. [44] (mean, 57) and Boileau et al. [45] (mean, 55.8). Improvement in active forward flexion also occurred across studies: Wall et al. [14] (from 86° to 137°), Sersohn et al. [43] (from 56° to 121°), Boileau et al. [3] (from 82° to 123°), Muilieri et al. [46] (from 53° to 134°), and Levy et al. [47] (from 38° to 72°). A long-term study by Molé and Favard with at least 10 years follow-up [35] demonstrated that 89 % of prostheses were still in place, and 72 % of the patients had a Constant score greater than 30 points. Radiographic deterioration, however, started to appear after 5–6 years, and clinical deterioration appeared after approximately 8 years.

Patients with rheumatoid arthritis and adequate glenoid bone stock have encouraging short-term results, showing good pain relief and significant improvement in Constant score [48–50]. Studies with follow-up between 5 and 10 years suggest faster radiographic deterioration than in rotator cuff disease [51]. However, a higher rate of infection is found in this group [48, 49].

Acute three- and four-part proximal humerus fractures in the elderly have been successfully treated by RTSA [52, 53]. Hemiarthroplasty has long been the "gold standard" in these fractures in which the risk of nonunion, malunion, implant failure, or osteonecrosis precludes fragment fixation [54–56]. The repair and healing of the greater and lesser tuberosities have the greatest impact on clinical outcomes in hemiarthroplasty [57–60]. In contrast, RTSA relies less on a functioning rotator cuff and/or tuberosity healing than hemiarthroplasty does. In the first systematic review to date comparing hemiarthroplasty and RTSA for the treatment of acute fractures, Namdari [61] found similar functional outcomes and physical examination parameters between the groups. Clinical complications differed substantially, however, with a four times greater odds of complication after RTSA. Less optimal results than those achieved in the treatment of cuff tear arthropathy may be expected. Postoperative abduction between 90° and 100° has been reported, with significant variation in external rotation and poor internal rotation [42, 62–64].

Revision surgery with RTSA can be plagued by complications and results are inferior to those obtained for other indications [14, 65]. Furthermore, studies have shown limited gains in range of movement and pain relief and minimal gain or even worsening of rotation [3, 14, 47, 63, 66]. Revising failed hemiarthroplasty to RTSA has resulted in a complication rate between 32 and 50 % depending on the study [14, 65]. Failed total shoulder arthroplasty revision surgery can yield acceptable functional results, but primary total shoulder arthroplasty results are consistently better [67]. Wall et al. [14] found that patients who received primary RTSA for failed arthroplasty or posttraumatic arthritis had worse results and more complications than patients who received RTSA for cuff tear arthropathy, osteoarthritis with cuff tear, and massive cuff tear. A thorough risk-benefit analysis must be assessed for patients after failed proximal humerus fractures because RTSA is the only surgical procedure that will restore overhead function [4].

There are few studies of revisions of failed RTSA. Boileau et al. [68] recently examined a series of revisions and found that, similar to previous reports instability, humeral complications (aseptic loosening, implant derotation, and fractures), and infection were the most common complications requiring surgical reintervention [14, 25, 40, 66, 69–72]. Outcomes were encouraging, with preservation of shoulder function, a mean Constant score of 47 points compared with

58 points in a previous series of primary RSA [45], and 89 % of the patients were satisfied. It is clear that revision surgery of a failed or complicated RTSA is a high-risk surgery since 30 % of the patients in this series had complications that required further surgical interventions.

Although the majority of RTSA are performed in the older patient population, it is becoming more commonplace in individuals younger than 60. There are few studies on this younger demographic population, however. Findings from a recent retrospective study of 41 patients aged younger than 65 by Ek et al. [44] show that RTSA in younger patients provides subjective improvement of overall shoulder function maintained up to 10 years after treatment. There was a high complication rate of 37.5 % and implant survivorship was only 75 %. Dillon et al. [73] recently completed a multicenter retrospective cohort study on shoulder arthroplasty in 504 patients aged 59 years or younger versus 2,477 patients aged 60 years or older, with a mean follow-up of 2.2 years. There was a two times higher risk of revision arthroplasty in the younger cohort at early follow-up. In their study of patients aged <60 years with RTSA, Sersohn et al. [43] reported a Constant score of 54.3, complication rate of 13.9 %, and implant survivorship of 91 % at a mean follow-up of 2.8 years. In a study of RTSA patients with a mean age of 52.2 years and mean follow-up of 36.5 months, Muh et al. [74] reported excellent improvement in active forward elevation (from 54.6° to 134.0°); however, overall satisfaction was 81 %, which is substantially lower than rates for older patients reported in the literature (90–96 %) [35, 40].

As RTSAs are performed on younger patients, long-term implant survivorship becomes particularly crucial. Unfortunately, there is a paucity of literature on this long-term data. A recent multicenter analysis of 489 patients with massive cuff tears with or without glenohumeral arthropathy who underwent RTSA by Favard et al. [75] determined complication rates, functional scores over time, survivorship, and whether radiographs would develop signs of loosening. There was a complication rate of 22 %. Survivorship free of revision was 89 % at 10 years with a marked break occurring at 2 and 9 years. Survivorship to a Constant score of less than 30 was 72 % at 10 years with a noticeable break at 8 years. Progressive radiographic changes were apparent after 5 years, and there was an increasing frequency of large notches with long-term follow-up. Based on these findings, the authors concluded that on average, there is a progressive decline in patient function after the eighth year the authors urge caution when indicating RTSA, especially in younger patients.

Complications

Drawing definitive conclusions regarding complications in RTSA is sometimes difficult because of heterogeneity in reporting studies, but salient trends exist in the literature. In general, previous surgery is a risk factor for increased complications [14], reoperations [25], and lower implant survival rates [24].

Scapular notching, erosion of the scapular neck related to impingement by the medial rim of the humeral cup during adduction, is one of the most common complications in many reports [12, 25, 40, 76–79] (Fig. 10.10). In a large multicenter trial comprised of 461 shoulders, Lévigne

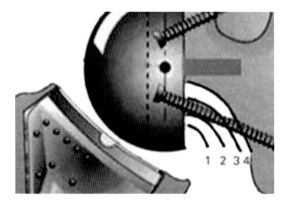

Fig. 10.10 A drawing shows classification of scapular notching according to Sirveaux et al. [39]. Grade *1* shows a notch limited to the scapular pillar, Grade *2* shows a notch reaching the inferior screw of the base plate, Grade *3* shows a notch extending beyond the inferior screw, and Grade *4* shows a notch reaching the base plate's central peg

et al. [80] found an incidence of 68 % at a mean follow-up of 51 months. Furthermore, they demonstrated that notching was accompanied by decreases in strength and anterior elevation as well as an increased incidence in humeral and glenoid radiolucent lines. Inferior placement of the baseplate on the glenoid plate has been shown by Nyffeler et al. [32] to prevent the occurrence of notching and also improve range of motion. Glenospheres with a lateral center of rotation have been shown to produce lower rates of scapular notching [81–83].

In cuff tear arthropathy, the dislocation rate has been reported to be between 2 and 3.4 % [35, 50, 84]. Instability is almost always anterior, but the reasons are not well known. Correct deltoid tension and correct component version are necessary for stability [53]. Dislocation within the first 3 months is most likely due to technical error, and closed reduction is usually not successful. On the other hand, a late dislocation (>1 year postoperatively) has a higher likelihood of a successful closed reduction [35].

The incidence of deep infection in primary RTSA was 4 and 5.4 % in two studies [35, 50], compared with 1.1 % for anatomic replacement [85]. Infection rates are even higher with revision surgery [3, 25]. RTSA may be susceptible to infection because of the large subacromial dead space created by the inverse prosthesis [4]. The two most common organisms responsible for infections after shoulder surgery are *Propionibacterium acnes* and *Staphylococci*, which are mainly coagulase-negative [86]. Since component removal after RTSA can cause significant bone loss, some authors have advocated that patients with a deep infection should be managed with an initial irrigation and debridement, culture-driven intravenous antibiotics, and component retention [87].

Intraoperative glenoid complications are rare but they can occur because there is often erosion and medialization of the glenoid, leaving little bone stock for fixation. Glenoid loosening has been reported in 4.1 % of prostheses followed for longer than 2 years [35]. Treatment involves a staged procedure to fill the glenoid cavity with

Table 10.3 Complications

Scapular notching
Dislocation
Infection
Glenoid loosening
Acromion fracture
Humeral disassembly
Humeral fracture
Neuropraxia

autogenous bone and await incorporation with a hemiarthroplasty prior to reimplantation of the glenosphere.

Acromion fracture or even scapula spine fracture is another postoperative complication. Insufficiency fractures are characteristic and may result from overtensioning the deltoid [12], but the exact mechanism is poorly understood [25, 81, 88]. Postoperative fractures have been observed in 1.4–4 % of patients [50, 84]. The fracture usually occurs either through the acromion or at the base of the spine of the scapula [89, 90]. Despite causing minimal pain, the functional score and subjective satisfaction are reduced in patients who sustain acromial fractures [84, 91]. Treatment options are limited because there is little remaining bone for fixation. Preoperative acromial fragmentation due to cuff tear arthropathy or os acromiale, however, is not a contraindication to RTSA because no adverse effects on outcome have been observed [89] (Table 10.3).

Conclusions

Prior to the advent of RTSA, cuff tear arthropathy was a severely debilitating condition with few options. While imperfections still exist, modern RTSA has proven to be an extremely successful innovation in the treatment of this disease. Although sophisticated implants and advanced surgical techniques have expanded indications for RTSA, validation from well-designed long-term studies will help guide its future implementation in cuff tear arthropathy and other pathological conditions of the shoulder.

References

1. Basamania CJ. Hemiarthroplasty for cuff tear arthropathy. In: Advanced reconstruction shoulder. Rosemont: American Academy of Orthopaedic Surgeons; 2007. p. 567–78.
2. Rockwood CA. The reverse total shoulder prosthesis. The new kid on the block. J Bone Joint Surg Am. 2007;89(2):233–5. doi:10.2106/JBJS.F.01394.
3. Boileau P, Watkinson D, Hatzidakis AM, Hovorka I. Neer Award 2005: the Grammont reverse shoulder prosthesis: results in cuff tear arthritis, fracture sequelae, and revision arthroplasty. J Shoulder Elbow Surg. 2006;15(5):527–40. doi:10.1016/j.jse.2006.01.003.
4. Gerber C, Pennington SD, Nyffeler RW. Reverse total shoulder arthroplasty. J Am Acad Orthop Surg. 2009;17(5):284–95.
5. Grammont P, Trouilloud P, Laffay JP, Deries X. Study and realization of a new shoulder prosthesis [in French]. Rhumatologie. 1987;39:17–22.
6. McCarty DJ, Halverson PB, Carrera GF, Brewer BJ, Kozin F. "Milwaukee shoulder" – association of microspheroids containing hydroxyapatite crystals, active collagenase, and neutral protease with rotator cuff defects. I Clinical aspects. Arthritis Rheum. 1981;24(3):464–73. Available at: http://eutils.ncbi.nlm.nih.gov/entrez/eutils/elink.fcgi?dbfrom=pubmed&id=6260120&retmode=ref&cmd=prlinks.
7. Neer CS, Craig EV, Fukuda H. Cuff-tear arthropathy. J Bone Joint Surg Am. 1983;65(9):1232–44.
8. Nam D, Kepler CK, Neviaser AS, et al. Reverse total shoulder arthroplasty: current concepts, results, and component wear analysis. J Bone Joint Surg. 2010;92 Suppl 2:23–35. doi:10.2106/JBJS.J.00769.
9. Edwards TB, Boulahia A, Kempf J-F, Boileau P, Nemoz C, Walch G. The influence of rotator cuff disease on the results of shoulder arthroplasty for primary osteoarthritis: results of a multicenter study. J Bone Joint Surg Am. 2002;84-A(12):2240–8.
10. Sanchez-Sotelo J, Cofield RH, Rowland CM. Shoulder hemiarthroplasty for glenohumeral arthritis associated with severe rotator cuff deficiency. J Bone Joint Surg Am. 2001;83-A(12):1814–22.
11. Sanchez-Sotelo J. Reverse total shoulder arthroplasty. Clin Anat. 2009;22(2):172–82. doi:10.1002/ca.20736.
12. Boileau P, Watkinson DJ, Hatzidakis AM, Balg F. Grammont reverse prosthesis: design, rationale, and biomechanics. J Shoulder Elbow Surg. 2005;14(1 Suppl S):147S–61.
13. Gartsman GM, Edwards TB, editors. Shoulder arthroplasty. 1st ed. Philadelphia: Saunders; 2008.
14. Wall B, Nové-Josserand L, O'Connor DP, Edwards TB, Walch G. Reverse total shoulder arthroplasty: a review of results according to etiology. J Bone Joint Surg Am. 2007;89(7):1476–85. doi:10.2106/JBJS.F.00666.
15. Williams GR, Rockwood CA. Hemiarthroplasty in rotator cuff-deficient shoulders. J Shoulder Elbow Surg. 1996;5(5):362–7.

16. Amstutz HC, Thomas BJ, Kabo JM, Jinnah RH, Dorey FJ. The Dana total shoulder arthroplasty. J Bone Joint Surg Am. 1988;70(8):1174–82.

17. Figgie MP, Inglis AE, Figgie HE, Sobel M, Burstein AH, Kraay MJ. Custom total shoulder arthroplasty in inflammatory arthritis. Preliminary results. J Arthroplasty. 1992;7(1):1–6.

18. Neer CS, Watson KC, Stanton FJ. Recent experience in total shoulder replacement. J Bone Joint Surg Am. 1982;64(3):319–37.

19. Raiss P, Aldinger PR, Kasten P, Rickert M, Loew M. Total shoulder replacement in young and middle-aged patients with glenohumeral osteoarthritis. J Bone Joint Surg Br. 2008;90(6):764–9. doi:10.1302/0301-620X.90B6.20387.

20. Yian EH, Werner CML, Nyffeler RW, et al. Radiographic and computed tomography analysis of cemented pegged polyethylene glenoid components in total shoulder replacement. J Bone Joint Surg Am. 2005;87(9):1928–36. doi:10.2106/JBJS.D.02675.

21. Ecklund KJ, Lee TQ, Tibone J, Gupta R. Rotator cuff tear arthropathy. J Am Acad Orthop Surg. 2007;15(6):340–9.

22. Feeley BT, Gallo RA, Craig EV. Cuff tear arthropathy: current trends in diagnosis and surgical management. J Shoulder Elbow Surg. 2009;18(3):484–94. doi:10.1016/j.jse.2008.11.003.

23. Boileau P, Baqué F, Valerio L, Ahrens P, Chuinard C, Trojani C. Isolated arthroscopic biceps tenotomy or tenodesis improves symptoms in patients with massive irreparable rotator cuff tears. J Bone Joint Surg Am. 2007;89(4):747–57. doi:10.2106/JBJS.E.01097.

24. Guery J, Favard L, Sirveaux F, Oudet D, Molé D, Walch G. Reverse total shoulder arthroplasty. Survivorship analysis of eighty replacements followed for five to ten years. J Bone Joint Surg Am. 2006;88(8):1742–7. doi:10.2106/JBJS.E.00851.

25. Werner CML, Steinmann PA, Gilbart M, Gerber C. Treatment of painful pseudoparesis due to irreparable rotator cuff dysfunction with the Delta III reverse-ball-and-socket total shoulder prosthesis. J Bone Joint Surg Am. 2005;87(7):1476–86. doi:10.2106/JBJS.D.02342.

26. Frankle M, Levy JC, Pupello D, et al. The reverse shoulder prosthesis for glenohumeral arthritis associated with severe rotator cuff deficiency: a minimum two-year follow-up study of sixty patients surgical technique. J Bone Joint Surg Am. 2006;88(Suppl 1 Pt 2):178–90. doi:10.2106/JBJS.F.00123.

27. Gerber C, Pennington SD, Lingenfelter EJ, Sukthankar A. Reverse Delta-III total shoulder replacement combined with latissimus dorsi transfer: a preliminary report. J Bone Joint Surg Am. 2007;89(5):940–7.

28. Favre P, Loeb MD, Helmy N, Gerber C. Latissimus dorsi transfer to restore external rotation with reverse shoulder arthroplasty: a biomechanical study. J Shoulder Elbow Surg. 2008;17(4):650–8. doi:10.1016/j.jse.2007.12.010.

29. Boileau P, Chuinard C, Roussanne Y, Bicknell RT. Reverse shoulder arthroplasty combined with a modified latissimus dorsi and teres major tendon transfer for shoulder pseudoparalysis associated with dropping arm. Clin Orthop Relat Res. 2008;466(3):584–93.

30. Gulotta LV, Choi D, Marinello P, et al. Anterior deltoid deficiency in reverse total shoulder replacement: a biomechanical study with cadavers. J Bone Joint Surg Br. 2012;94(12):1666–9.

31. Kölbel R, Friedebold G. Stabilization of shoulders with bone and muscle defects using joint replacement implants. In: Shoulder surgery. At Louis: Mosby; 1984.

32. Nyffeler RW, Werner CML, Gerber C. Biomechanical relevance of glenoid component positioning in the reverse Delta III total shoulder prosthesis. J Shoulder Elbow Surg. 2005;14(5):524–8. doi:10.1016/j.jse.2004.09.010.

33. Swanson AB, de Groot Swanson G, Sattel AB, Cendo RD, Hynes D, Jar-Ning W. Bipolar implant shoulder arthroplasty. Long-term results. Clin Orthop Relat Res. 1989;249:227–47.

34. Boulahia A, Edwards TB, Walch G, Baratta RV. Early results of a reverse design prosthesis in the treatment of arthritis of the shoulder in elderly patients with a large rotator cuff tear. Orthopedics. 2002;25(2):129–33.

35. Mole D, Favard L. Excentered scapulohumeral osteoarthritis. Rev Chir Orthop Reparatrice Appar Mot. 2007;93(6 Suppl):37–94.

36. Clark J, Ritchie J, Song F, Kissenberth M, Tolan S, Hart N, Hawkins R. Complication rates, dislocation, pain, and postoperative range of motion after reverse shoulder arthroplasty in patients with and without repair of the subscapularis. J Shoulder Elbow Surg. 2012;21(1):36–41.

37. Gulotta LV, Choi D, Marinello P, et al. Humeral component retroversion in reverse total shoulder arthroplasty: a biomechanical study. J Shoulder Elbow Surg. 2012;9:1121–7. doi:10.1016/j.jse.2011.07.027.

38. Gutiérrez S, Comiskey CA, Luo Z-P, Pupello DR, Frankle MA. Range of impingement-free abduction and adduction deficit after reverse shoulder arthroplasty. Hierarchy of surgical and implant-design-related factors. J Bone Joint Surg Am. 2008;90(12):2606–15. doi:10.2106/JBJS.H.00012.

39. Simovitch RW, Zumstein MA, Lohri E, Helmy N, Gerber C. Predictors of scapular notching in patients managed with the Delta III reverse total shoulder replacement. J Bone Joint Surg Am. 2007;89(3):588–600. doi:10.2106/JBJS.F.00226.

40. Sirveaux F, Favard L, Oudet D, Huquet D, Walch G, Mole D. Grammont inverted total shoulder arthroplasty in the treatment of glenohumeral osteoarthritis with massive rupture of the cuff. Results of a multicentre study of 80 shoulders. J Bone Joint Surg Br. 2004;86(3):388–95.

41. Gerber C, Vinh TS, Hertel R, Hess CW. Latissimus dorsi transfer for the treatment of massive tears of the rotator cuff. A preliminary report. Clin Orthop Relat Res. 1988;232:51–61.

42. Young SW, Zhu M, Walker CG, Poon PC. Comparison of functional outcomes of reverse shoulder arthroplasty with those of hemiarthroplasty in the treatment of cuff-tear arthropathy: a matched-pair analysis. J Bone Joint Surg Am. 2013;95(10):910–5.

43. Sershon RA, Van Thiel GS, Lin EC, et al. Clinical outcomes of reverse total shoulder arthroplasty in patients aged younger than 60 years. J Shoulder Elbow Surg. 2013. doi:10.1016/j.jse.2013.07.047.

44. Ek ETH, Neukom L, Catanzaro S, Gerber C. Reverse total shoulder arthroplasty for massive irreparable rotator cuff tears in patients younger than 65 years old: results after five to fifteen years. J Shoulder Elbow Surg. 2013;22(9):1199–208. doi:10.1016/j.jse.2012.11.016.

45. Boileau P, Gonzalez J-F, Chuinard C, Bicknell R, Walch G. Reverse total shoulder arthroplasty after failed rotator cuff surgery. J Shoulder Elbow Surg. 2009;18(4):600–6. doi:10.1016/j.jse.2009.03.011.

46. Mulieri P, Dunning P, Klein S, Pupello D. Reverse shoulder arthroplasty for the treatment of irreparable rotator cuff tear without glenohumeral arthritis. J Bone Joint Surg Am. 2010;92(15):2544–56.

47. Levy J, Frankle M, Mighell M, Pupello D. The use of the reverse shoulder prosthesis for the treatment of failed hemiarthroplasty for proximal humeral fracture. J Bone Joint Surg Am. 2007;89(2):292–300. doi:10.2106/JBJS.E.01310.

48. Rittmeister M, Kerschbaumer F. Grammont reverse total shoulder arthroplasty in patients with rheumatoid arthritis and nonreconstructible rotator cuff lesions. J Shoulder Elbow Surg. 2001;10(1):17–22. doi:10.1067/mse.2001.110515.

49. Holcomb JO, Herbert D, Mighell M, et al. Reverse shoulder arthroplasty in patients with rheumatoid arthritis. J Shoulder Elbow Surg. 2010;19(7):1076–84. doi:10.1016/j.jse.2009.11.049.

50. Nolan BM, Ankerson E, Wiater JM. Reverse total shoulder arthroplasty improves function in cuff tear arthropathy. Clin Orthop Relat Res. 2011;469(9):2476–82. doi:10.1007/s11999-010-1683-z.

51. Woodruff MJ, Cohen AP, Bradley JG. Arthroplasty of the shoulder in rheumatoid arthritis with rotator cuff dysfunction. Int Orthop. 2003;27(1):7–10. doi:10.1007/s00264-002-0406-9.

52. Sirveaux F, Navez G, Favard L, Boileau P, Walch G, Mole D. Reverse prosthesis for acute proximal humerus fracture: the multicenter study. In: Reverse shoulder arthroplasty: clinical results, complications, revision. Montpellier: Sauramps Medical; 2006. p. 73–80.

53. Matsen FA, Boileau P, Walch G, Gerber C, Bicknell RT. The reverse total shoulder arthroplasty. J Bone Joint Surg Am. 2007;89(3):660–7.

54. Neer CS. Articular replacement for the humeral head. J Bone Joint Surg Am. 1955;37-A(2):215–28.

55. Zyto K, Wallace WA, Frostick SP, Preston BJ. Outcome after hemiarthroplasty for three- and four-part fractures of the proximal humerus. J Shoulder Elbow Surg. 1998;7(2):85–9.

56. Goldman RT, Koval KJ, Cuomo F, Gallagher MA, Zuckerman JD. Functional outcome after humeral head replacement for acute three- and four-part proximal humeral fractures. J Shoulder Elbow Surg. 1995;4(2):81–6.

57. Boileau P, Krishnan SG, Tinsi L, Walch G, Coste JS, Mole D. Tuberosity malposition and migration: reasons for poor outcomes after hemiarthroplasty for displaced fractures of the proximal humerus. J Shoulder Elbow Surg. 2002;11(5):401–12.

58. Kralinger F, Schwaiger R, Wambacher M, et al. Outcome after primary hemiarthroplasty for fracture of the head of the humerus. A retrospective multicentre study of 167 patients. J Bone Joint Surg Br. 2004;86(2):217–9.

59. Krishnan SG, Reineck JR, Bennion PD, Feher L, Burkhead WZ. Shoulder arthroplasty for fracture: does a fracture-specific stem make a difference? Clin Orthop Relat Res. 2011;469(12):3317–23. doi:10.1007/s11999-011-1919-6.

60. Reuther F, Mühlhäusler B, Wahl D, Nijs S. Functional outcome of shoulder hemiarthroplasty for fractures: a multicentre analysis. Injury. 2010;41(6):606–12. doi:10.1016/j.injury.2009.11.019.

61. Namdari S, Horneff JG, Baldwin K. Comparison of hemiarthroplasty and reverse arthroplasty for treatment of proximal humeral fractures: a systematic review. J Bone Joint Surg Am. 2013;95(18):1701–8. doi:10.2106/JBJS.L.01115.

62. Bufquin T, Hersan A, Hubert L, Massin P. Reverse shoulder arthroplasty for the treatment of three- and four-part fractures of the proximal humerus in the elderly: a prospective review of 43 cases with a short-term follow-up. J Bone Joint Surg Br. 2007;89(4):516–20. doi:10.1302/0301-620X.89B4.18435.

63. Flury MP, Frey P, Goldhahn J, Schwyzer H-K, Simmen BR. Reverse shoulder arthroplasty as a salvage procedure for failed conventional shoulder replacement due to cuff failure – midterm results. Int Orthop. 2011;35(1):53–60. doi:10.1007/s00264-010-0990-z.

64. Klein M, Juschka M, Hinkenjann B, Scherger B, Ostermann PAW. Treatment of comminuted fractures of the proximal humerus in elderly patients with the Delta III reverse shoulder prosthesis. J Orthop Trauma. 2008;22(10):698–704. doi:10.1097/BOT.0b013e31818afe40.

65. Walch G, Boileau P, Mole D, Favard L, Levigne C, Sirveaux F, editors. Reverse shoulder arthroplasty: clinical results, complications, revision. In: Revision of shoulder hemiarthroplasty with reverse prosthesis. Sauramps Medical, Montpellier; 2006. p. 217–28.

66. Holcomb JO, Cuff D, Petersen SA, Pupello DR, Frankle MA. Revision reverse shoulder arthroplasty for glenoid baseplate failure after primary reverse shoulder arthroplasty. J Shoulder Elbow Surg. 2009;18(5):717–23. doi:10.1016/j.jse.2008.11.017.

67. Walch G, Mole D, Mole, et al., editors. Reverse shoulder arthroplasty: clinical results, complications, revision. In: The reverse shoulder prosthesis for revision of

failed total shoulder arthroplasty. Sauramps Medical, Montpellier; 2006. p. 231–42.

68. Boileau P, Melis B, Duperron D, Moineau G, Rumian AP, Han Y. Revision surgery of reverse shoulder arthroplasty. J Shoulder Elbow Surg. 2013;22(10): 1359–70. doi:10.1016/j.jse.2013.02.004.

69. Cuff D, Levy JC, Gutiérrez S, Frankle MA. Torsional stability of modular and non-modular reverse shoulder humeral components in a proximal humeral bone loss model. J Shoulder Elbow Surg. 2011;20(4):646–51. doi:10.1016/j.jse.2010.10.026.

70. Edwards TB, Williams MD, Labriola JE, Elkousy HA, Gartsman GM, O'Connor DP. Subscapularis insufficiency and the risk of shoulder dislocation after reverse shoulder arthroplasty. J Shoulder Elbow Surg. 2009;18(6):892–6. doi:10.1016/j.jse.2008.12.013.

71. Lädermann A, Williams MD, Melis B, Hoffmeyer P, Walch G. Objective evaluation of lengthening in reverse shoulder arthroplasty. J Shoulder Elbow Surg. 2009;18(4):588–95. doi:10.1016/j.jse.2009.03.012.

72. Zumstein MA, Pinedo M, Old J, Boileau P. Problems, complications, reoperations, and revisions in reverse total shoulder arthroplasty: a systematic review. J Shoulder Elbow Surg. 2011;20(1): 146–57. doi:10.1016/j.jse.2010.08.001.

73. Dillon MT, Inacio MCS, Burke MF, Navarro RA, Yian EH. Shoulder arthroplasty in patients 59 years of age and younger. J Shoulder Elbow Surg. 2013;22(10): 1338–44. doi:10.1016/j.jse.2013.01.029.

74. Muh SJ, Streit JJ, Wanner JP, Lenarz CJ. Early follow-up of reverse total shoulder arthroplasty in patients sixty years of age or younger. J Bone Joint Surg Am. 2013;95(20):1877–83.

75. Favard L, Levigne C, Nerot C, Gerber C, De Wilde L, Molé D. Reverse prostheses in arthropathies with cuff tear: are survivorship and function maintained over time? Clin Orthop Relat Res. 2011;469(9):2469–75. doi:10.1007/s11999-011-1833-y.

76. Grassi FA, Murena L, Valli F, Alberio R. Six-year experience with the Delta III reverse shoulder prosthesis. J Orthop Surg (Hong Kong). 2009;17(2):151–6. Available at: http://eutils.ncbi.nlm.nih.gov/entrez/eutils/elink.fcgi?dbfrom=pubmed&id=19721141&retmode=ref&cmd=prlinks.

77. John M, Pap G, Angst F, et al. Short-term results after reversed shoulder arthroplasty (Delta III) in patients with rheumatoid arthritis and irreparable rotator cuff tear. Int Orthop. 2010;34(1):71–7. doi:10.1007/s00264-009-0733-1.

78. Farshad M, Gerber C. Reverse total shoulder arthroplasty-from the most to the least common complication. Int Orthop. 2010;34(8):1075–82. doi:10.1007/s00264-010-1125-2.

79. Vanhove B, Beugnies A. Grammont's reverse shoulder prosthesis for rotator cuff arthropathy. A retrospective study of 32 cases. Acta Orthop Belg. 2004;70(3):219–25.

80. Levigne C, Garret J, Boileau P, Alami G, Favard L, Walch G. Scapular notching in reverse shoulder arthroplasty: is it important to avoid it and how? Clin Orthop Relat Res. 2011;469(9):2512–20.

81. Levy JC, Virani N, Pupello D, Frankle M. Use of the reverse shoulder prosthesis for the treatment of failed hemiarthroplasty in patients with glenohumeral arthritis and rotator cuff deficiency. J Bone Joint Surg Br. 2007;89(2):189–95. doi:10.1302/0301-620X.89B2.18161.

82. Cuff D, Pupello D, Virani N, Levy J, Frankle M. Reverse shoulder arthroplasty for the treatment of rotator cuff deficiency. J Bone Joint Surg Am. 2008;90(6):1244–51. doi:10.2106/JBJS.G.00775.

83. Kalouche I, Sevivas N, Wahegaonker A, Sauzières P, Katz D, Valenti P. Reverse shoulder arthroplasty: does reduced medialisation improve radiological and clinical results? Acta Orthop Belg. 2009;75(2):158–66. Available at: http://eutils.ncbi.nlm.nih.gov/entrez/eutils/elink.fcgi?dbfrom=pubmed&id=19492554&retmode=ref&cmd=prlinks.

84. Naveed MA, Kitson J, Bunker TD. The Delta III reverse shoulder replacement for cuff tear arthropathy: a single-centre study of 50 consecutive procedures. J Bone Joint Surg Br. 2011;93(1):57–61. doi:10.1302/0301-620X.93B1.24218.

85. Gonzalez J-F, Alami GB, Baqué F, Walch G, Boileau P. Complications of unconstrained shoulder prostheses. J Shoulder Elbow Surg. 2011;20(4):666–82. doi:10.1016/j.jse.2010.11.017.

86. Dodson CC, Thomas A, Dines JS, Nho SJ, Williams RJ, Altchek DW. Medial ulnar collateral ligament reconstruction of the elbow in throwing athletes. Am J Sports Med. 2006;34(12):1926–32. doi:10.1177/0363546506290988.

87. Zavala JA, Clark JC, Kissenberth MJ, Tolan SJ, Hawkins RJ. Management of deep infection after reverse total shoulder arthroplasty: a case series. J Shoulder Elbow Surg. 2012;21(10):1310–5. doi:10.1016/j.jse.2011.08.047.

88. Sarris IK, Papadimitriou NG, Sotereanos DG. Bipolar hemiarthroplasty for chronic rotator cuff tear arthropathy. J Arthroplasty. 2003;18(2):169–73. doi:10.1054/arth.2003.50041.

89. Walch G, Mottier F, Wall B, Boileau P, Molé D, Favard L. Acromial insufficiency in reverse shoulder arthroplasties. J Shoulder Elbow Surg. 2009;18(3): 495–502. doi:10.1016/j.jse.2008.12.002.

90. Wahlquist TC, Hunt AF, Braman JP. Acromial base fractures after reverse total shoulder arthroplasty: report of five cases. J Shoulder Elbow Surg. 2011;20(7):1178–83. doi:10.1016/j.jse.2011.01.029.

91. Walch G, Young AA, Boileau P, Loew M, Gazielly D, Molé D. Patterns of loosening of polyethylene keeled glenoid components after shoulder arthroplasty for primary osteoarthritis: results of a multicenter study with more than five years of follow-up. J Bone Joint Surg Am. 2012;94:145–50. doi:10.2106/JBJS.J.00699.

Treatment Algorithm for Patients with Massive Rotator Cuff Tears

11

Brian Grawe and Lawrence V. Gulotta

Pearls and Pitfalls

Pearls
- Local anesthetic injection (subacromial space) can provide key diagnostic information to discern motion limited secondary to pain from those with true pseudoparalysis.
- Anterior deltoid strengthening is the key to nonoperative management.
- Maintenance of CA arch is a must during arthroscopic management.
- Patients must be counseled that following arthroscopic treatment, their strength will increase only in so much that it was being limited by pain preoperatively.
- Ideal candidates for latissimus dorsi tendon transfer must have an intact subscapularis, without concomitant glenohumeral arthritis.
- The use of scaffolds in the treatment of irreparable rotator cuff tears must be approached cautiously as little clinical evidence supports their widespread use.
- Hemiarthroplasty can provide reliable pain relief and is best utilized in patients who have maintained elevation.
- Reverse shoulder arthroplasty should be reserved for patients with irreparable tears of the rotator cuff and pseudoparalysis of the shoulder.
- Tailor the treatment plan based on individual's symptoms and physical exam findings.

Pitfalls
- The benefit of nonoperative treatment modalities may not persist with time.
- Violation of the CA arch during arthroscopic treatment may lead to late anterosuperior escape of the humeral head.
- Outcomes following tendon transfers will be limited if patients are not prepared for the prolonged rehabilitation that is required.
- Hemiarthroplasty should not be performed in patients who already have anterosuperior escape of the humeral head.
- Reverse shoulder arthroplasty has shown early promising clinical results; however, the technique has a relatively steep learning curve and the long-term results are unclear.

B. Grawe, MD
Sports Medicine and Shoulder Service,
Hospital for Special Surgery, 535 E 70th Street,
New York, NY 10021, USA

L.V. Gulotta, MD (✉)
Sports Medicine and Shoulder Service,
Hospital for Special Surgery, 535 E 70th Street,
New York, NY 10021, USA

Department of Orthopedic Surgery, Weill Cornell
Medical School, New York, NY, USA
e-mail: GulottaL@hss.edu

L.V. Gulotta and E.V. Craig (eds.), *Massive Rotator Cuff Tears: Diagnosis and Management*,
DOI 10.1007/978-1-4899-7494-5_11, © Springer Science+Business Media New York 2015

Introduction

Massive and irreparable tears of the rotator cuff represent a complex clinical spectrum that challenges even the most experienced clinician. Consensus regarding optimal treatment of an irreparable rotator cuff tear is lacking, and often an individualized approach to each patient and the existent pathology must be undertaken. Untreated rotator cuff tears often progress over time and commonly represent a collective source of pain and disability, especially in the elderly population. Often tears advance through concomitant fatty infiltration and tendon retraction, the presence of which makes repair technically difficult and subject to an unacceptably high failure rate. Tissue quality in such tears is frequently inelastic, leading to scaring and adhesion formation [1]. The unpredictable results following attempted repair often do not warrant the morbidity associated with immobilization, physical therapy, and missed time from work following surgery [2]. As a result, alternative treatment options have been developed to aid surgeons in the successful management of patients with irreparable tears of the rotator cuff.

The purpose of this chapter is to appraise and critically evaluate the anticipated outcomes for interventions in the setting of an irreparable tear of the rotator cuff. It must be noted that the terms massive rotator cuff tear and irreparable rotator cuff tear are not mutually exclusive. Irreparable tears represent a subset of rotator cuff pathology that should not be repaired based on lack of healing potential, rather than technical feasibility. Many massive tears will lack the clinical and radiographic attributes outlined in this chapter and therefore are amenable to repair. We advocate for anatomic repair of the rotator cuff whenever possible, and the treatment of those patients is out of the scope of this chapter. Nonetheless the information presented will be useful in providing a generalizable treatment algorithm that can be individualized depending on specific patient circumstances in the challenging scenario of an irreparable rotator cuff tear.

Definition and Classification

Various classification systems have been proposed for the purposes of adequately defining a massive tear of the rotator cuff [3]. Presently, there is no consensus surrounding the definition, and most authors take into account anatomic and functional characteristics of the tendon when attempting to define and classify massive tears of the rotator cuff [1]. Unfortunately, each method has its own intrinsic set of limitations. A tear in which the anteroposterior dimension exceeds 5 cm was defined as massive by Cofield [4]. Others have classified massive tears based on the amount of exposed humeral head [5] or tear pattern in conjunction with tendon mobility [6]. The two tendon rule was initially proposed by Gerber and colleagues, where a massive tear, by definition, must have detachment of at least two tendons [7]. This system may better correlate with function, prognosis, and surgical outcome [3].

The presence of a massive rotator cuff tear does not necessarily indicate that the tissue is irreparable. Rather, Warner and Parsons have suggested that tears in which direct repair of the native tendon cannot be achieved to the anatomic footprint on the humerus should be categorized as irreparable [8]. This definition accounts for the surgeon's ability to perform tissue mobilization and other conventional soft tissue releases. Such tears are often chronic in nature, resulting in attritional changes to both the rotator cuff tendon proper and the muscle belly unit [9]. Tendon to bone healing is then further impeded by relative hypovascularity and an impoverished biologic environment, providing a mechanism by which even some small chronic tears become protracted and irreparable.

Mechanics/Pathomechanics

An intact and physiologic rotator cuff provides a force couple with the deltoid musculature to allow for balanced and stable glenohumeral joint mechanics, allowing centralization of the humeral head within the glenoid fossa. Disruption to the integrity of the rotator cuff often leads to pathologic shoulder dysfunction and subsequent pain. Burkhart et al. championed the concept that the rotator cuff functions as a unit much like a "suspension bridge" [10]. Specifically, the transverse plane of the glenohumeral joint is balanced by the interaction of the subscapularis tendon and the infraspinatus/teres minor complex, while the coronal plane is balanced via the interaction of the deltoid and the rotator cuff inferior to the equator of the humeral head [1]. This concept is supported clinically in those patients who have maintained an adequate fulcrum for shoulder motion, despite the presence of a significant tear of the supraspinatus tendon and even with extension into the infraspinatus tendon. Massive cuff tears by nature (tearing of at least two tendons) may compromise this fulcrum and lead to pain and disability.

Clinical Presentation

History

Massive rotator cuff tears commonly occur in elderly patients [11, 12]. Patient presentation is variable. It is of utmost importance to determine the main reason for why the patient is seeking medical care. Patients will most commonly complain of pain, but some will complain of weakness either in conjunction or in the absence of pain. Whether the patient chiefly complains of pain or weakness is an important delineation since the treatment algorithm is different for each complaint.

Occasionally, patients will report an acute traumatic event that is associated with a loss of function, while others may describe a more insidious onset of symptoms and dysfunction. The clinician should not be quick to offer operative treatment for patients with an acute injury in which their imaging is most consistent with a chronic tear. Often, these patients have a good response to nonoperative treatment and may return to their baseline after the current insult subsides. Alternatively, some patients will sus-

tain an acute or chronic tear. The most common scenario is one where the patient has been coping well with a chronic tear of the supraspinatus and infraspinatus and then tears their subscapularis acutely and their shoulder decompensates. These patients may benefit from early surgical fixation of the acute portion of the tear in order to maximize function.

Physical Examination

A thorough physical examination of the patient's affected and non-affected shoulder plays a critical role in the diagnosis of a massive rotator cuff tear. The most important clinical exam finding is whether or not the patient can actively elevate their arm above horizontal. This is important since this information guides the treatment algorithm. Some patients are unable to elevate their arms due to pain inhibition and may not have true mechanical weakness. If there is any doubt, then an injection of local anesthetic in the subacromial space, with or without steroids, can be given and the patient's ability to elevate should be reexamined. If a patient is still unable to elevate following an injection, then that patient has true pseudoparalysis and their treatment should be tailored accordingly. For these patients, it is important to determine if they have anterosuperior escape. Patients with anterosuperior escape can still benefit from physical therapy, but its success is less predictable. Patients with anterosuperior escape often require reverse shoulder arthroplasty in order to restore elevation.

There are many telltale signs that can alert clinicians to the possibility of an irreparable tear. Key findings that may dictate later treatment options would be incompetence of the coracoacromial (CA) arch and significant deltoid atrophy. Violation of the coracoacromial arch leads to anterosuperior escape of the humeral head, whereas the outline of the humeral head will be grossly evident and visible on the anterior aspect of the involved shoulder. Marked atrophy of either the supra- or infraspinous fossae, on general inspection, can also suggest unreliable results if formal repair was to be considered.

A number of physical exam findings allude to likely irreparability and are consistently dependent upon the anatomic location of cuff tear. Massive rotator cuff tears will invariably affect the integrity of the supraspinatus tendon. Anterosuperior tears can frequently extend into the insertion of the subscapularis, whereas the more common posterosuperior tear pattern will extend into the footprints of the infraspinatus and teres minor tendons. Subscapularis involvement may reveal positive belly-press, lift-off, and bear-hug tests, along with an increase in passive external rotation [13]. Ascertainment of the relative size of posterosuperior tears can be accomplished primarily with two provocative maneuvers. A positive external rotation lag sign is often present when the infraspinatus tendon becomes incompetent [14], whereas a positive hornblower sign is more indicative of a larger tear involving the teres minor [15].

Imaging

Imaging studies will aid in clinical diagnosis of massive rotator cuff tears, while also allowing for the appropriate selection of available treatment options for those tears that are irreparable. Roentgenograms provide an effective first-line evaluation of the glenohumeral joint, acromion, and position of the humeral head. Massive tears are frequently associated with anterosuperior migration of the humeral head, thus demonstrating a decreased acromiohumeral interval (AHI). Predictable decreases of the AHI, as measured on a true anteroposterior radiograph of the shoulder, correlate well with tear size and progression [16]. Quantitatively, an AHI distance of less than 5 mm indicates a 2 tendon tear and should alert the surgeon that a likely massive tear of the rotator cuff is present. More recent studies have demonstrated correlation of the AHI and stage of fatty infiltration of the rotator cuff musculature, which has implication in terms of viability of an attempted tendon repair [17].

Magnetic resonance imaging (MRI) has recently evolved to become the gold standard for advanced imaging of the rotator cuff. It has the advantage of diagnosing tendon tears with excellent sensitivity and specificity [18]. MRI also allows for the accurate estimate of tear size, degree of tendon retraction, and fatty infiltration of the musculature [19]. As a result, MRI evaluation of rotator cuff tendon tears becomes especially useful when attempting to gauge reparability of the tear. Classically, the Goutallier system for grading and describing stages of fatty infiltration of the rotator cuff musculature has been accomplished with the aid of computed tomography [20]. Recently, this system has been adapted to MRI and subsequently correlated to surgical outcomes and retear rates [7, 21, 22]. Stages 3 and 4 fatty infiltration, as demonstrated on preoperative MRI, have been associated with no functional improvement after attempted repair [22]. With increasing fatty infiltration of greater than 50 %, it is accepted that tendon retearing with a paucity of healing will likely occur, even if tissue repair is technically feasible [2].

Ultrasound imaging has recently become an established modality for the evaluation and diagnosis of rotator cuff tendon tears. Its low cost and noninvasive nature make it a relatively appealing alternative to MRI; however, it is highly operator dependent and less reliable in assessing fatty infiltration of the muscle. Ultrasound also has the inability to penetrate the bone making the modality less useful when the tendon has retracted medial to the acromion. Consequently, ultrasound plays a limited role in the diagnostic work-up and evaluation of reparability of rotator cuff tears.

Treatment Options

Nonoperative

Physical therapy and the judicious utilization of steroid injections should represent the first-line treatment for massive tears of the rotator cuff. Functional improvement can be noted with activity modification and strengthening of the anterior deltoid. Secondary goals of physical therapy include muscle recruitment and reeducation, periscapular strengthening, and maintenance of glenohumeral motion. The basis of such programs is rooted in cadaveric biomechanical studies that demonstrate stable glenohumeral abduction, in the setting of a massive rotator cuff tear, through higher-force generation within the deltoid and remaining intact rotator cuff [23]. Numerous studies have demonstrated that patients with massive tears of the rotator cuff are still able to maintain adequate glenohumeral motion along with the ability to successfully perform activities of daily living [10, 24].

Ainsworth et al. described ten patients who underwent multimodal physical therapy for the treatment of an irreparable rotator cuff tear. After 12 weeks of therapy mean Oxford Shoulder Disability Questionnaire (OSDQ) scores improved 9 points, while Short Form-36 (SF-36) scores improved by 22 points. Therapy focused on patient education, posture correction, reeducation of muscle recruitment, stretching, strengthening, proprioception, and adaptation [25]. In a more specific anterior deltoid training program, Levy et al. were able to prospectively evaluate 17 patients with the clinical and radiographic diagnosis of an irreparable rotator cuff tear. Patients were assessed at a minimum of 9 months and their mean forward flexion improved 120°, and their mean Constant scores improved 34 points [26].

Arthroscopy

Debridement and Subacromial Decompression

Debridement of the torn rotator cuff tendons coupled with or without a subacromial decompression should be reserved as viable treatment options for the lower-demand and elderly patients. Great strides can be made in the way of pain relief, while improvements in strength and range of motion may only prove marginally [2]. This treatment option can also yield gains in patients who have maintained function of their shoulder, but are severely limited secondary to pain. Technical considerations focus on removal of pain generators – torn/degenerative edges of the rotator cuff and subacromial bursa – while

maintaining the coracoacromial (CA) arch. A limited acromioplasty can be performed, providing more space for the greater tuberosity. More recent attention has been turned to the reverse subacromial decompression, where the bare greater tuberosity is debrided to provide a more smooth acromiohumeral articulation during shoulder elevation (tuberoplasty) [27].

Partial Repair

Arthroscopic partial repair of a massive tear can yield successful results, when applied in the clinical setting of good remaining tissue quality. The goal of this technique is restoration of a stable glenohumeral fulcrum for shoulder activities, rather than complete closure of the tendon defect. The importance of recreating balanced kinematics in the shoulder joint was first recognized by Burkhart. He suggested that restoring the coronal force couple of the rotator cuff can yield reliable functional results in the face of an irreparable supraspinatus tear [28]. Aggressive treatment of infraspinatus tears and margin convergence sutures are techniques that can improve the mechanical advantage of the remaining intact rotator cuff.

Burkhart et al. demonstrated improved mean active forward flexion, 60° and 120° pre- and postoperatively, in 14 patients after partial repairs of massive tears [29]. These results were further supported by Duralde et al. who retrospectively reviewed the results of partial open repair of rotator cuff tears. Subjective and objective results were improved, with 92 % of patients reporting satisfaction with the outcome of their shoulder. All patients maintained good strength, while active elevation improved by a mean of 40° [30].

Biceps Tenotomy/Tenodesis

The precise function of the long head of the biceps remains largely unknown. In patients with massive rotator cuff tears, the tendon may theoretically function as a humeral head depressor, thus limiting superior escape of the humerus [31, 32]. Increasing clinical evidence now supports that the tendon offers minimal benefit to glenohumeral stability in patients with irreparable rotator cuff tears and likely functions solely as a pain generator. Electromyographic studies have demonstrated that the tendon's role is likely more passive than active and is quiescent during active shoulder abduction in the setting of massive rotator cuff tear [33].

Walch initially observed that patients with chronic rotator cuff insufficiency experienced pain relief after sustaining a senescent rupture of the long head of their biceps tendon [9]. Subsequently, he reported good long-term clinical results of isolated biceps tenotomy in patients with massive rotator cuff tears. Fatty infiltration of either the subscapularis or the teres minor was predictor of a worse outcome, and tenotomy did not affect the progression of glenohumeral osteoarthritis [34]. Other surgeons have confirmed these findings [35].

Suprascapular Nerve (SSN) Release

The relationship between pain and weakness associated with massive tears of the rotator cuff and neuropathy of the suprascapular nerve has garnered considerable attention over the recent years [36–38]. The suprascapular nerve, and its associated pathology, likely has two distinct mechanisms for causing pain and disability in the setting of rotator cuff pathology, the first being in the setting of repair. Warner et al. were able to demonstrate, via cadaveric studies, that lateral advancement of the supraspinatus and infraspinatus tendon of greater than 3 cm can produce excessive tension on the motor branches of the suprascapular nerve. This is a direct result of the nerve's close anatomic relationship to the bony floor of the supraspinatus fossa and its resultant tethering at the suprascapular notch. The authors theorized that tearing of the tendon and development of scar tissue place the nerve at further risk, and clinical failures associated with tendon mobilization might be due to nerve pathology [39]. In a similar fashion, massive posterosuperior tears can place excessive traction on the suprascapular nerve proper. Retraction of the muscle can directly lead to neuropathy, which may play a fundamental role in pain and weakness. This observation has recently been confirmed with the aid of electrodiagnostic studies (EMG) [40].

Boykin et al [36] showed EMG evidence of suprascapular neuropathy in 60 % of patients with a massive tear versus 30 % of those patients without a massive tear indicating a fairly high prevalence. However, it remains unclear if formal release at the suprascapular notch is necessary or if partial repair of the rotator cuff may take tension off of the nerve. Costouros et al. [38] demonstrated SSN reversal in six patients following partial or complete repair of massive rotator cuff tears.

Author's Preferred Use of Arthroscopy

Arthroscopy is indicated for patients with massive, irreparable tears who are able to elevate their arms. The primary purpose of this procedure is to reduce pain. Patients are told that their power will increase only in so much as it is limited by pain. At the time of surgery, an extensive debridement of all inflamed tissues is performed. A minimal acromioplasty is performed, but every effort is made to preserve the CA arch. If the long head of the biceps tendon is still present, it is tenotomized or tenodesed based on a preoperative conversation with the patient. When possible, a margin convergence repair of the rotator cuff is performed. The goal is a tension-free repair (Fig. 11.1). If the tension allows, then a single anchor is used to solidify the fixation to the bone. Suprascapular neuropathy is not routinely evaluated and release is not routinely performed. The goal of rehabilitation is pain-free active motion. The therapist is told not to expect significant gains in strength, and strengthening exercises that cause pain are avoided.

Tendon Transfers

Salvage reconstruction, with a muscle tendon transfer, is a feasible surgical option for an irreparable rotator cuff tear in patients who have primary symptoms which attribute to weakness, pain, and impaired active motion. Various techniques have been described for rotator cuff reconstruction that include local tendon transposition, distant tendon transfer, and muscle flap reconstruction.

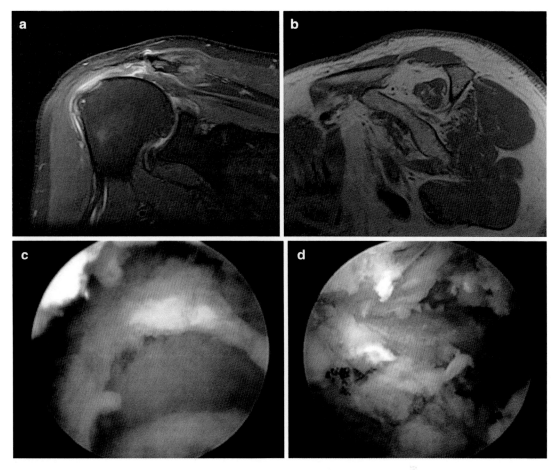

Fig. 11.1 Patient is a 75-year-old male with a 3-year history of shoulder pain without a defined traumatic event. He is able to elevate his arm above his head, but despite physical therapy and steroid injections, the pain continues to interfere with his quality of life. MRI in the coronal plan shows a tear of the supraspinatus with retraction almost to the glenoid and thinning of the tendon (**a**). Sagittal plan MRI shows atrophy of the supraspinatus and the infraspinatus (**b**). At the time of arthroscopy, the tendon was retracted and immobile (**c**). Therefore, a margin convergence-type repair was performed (**d**). Two years after surgery, the patient is pain free, though still has weakness with lifting objects away from his body

Donor tendon selection is grounded on a multitude of variables, but typically centers on location of the rotator cuff tear and the specific functional deficits the patient is experiencing. Common tendons utilized include the latissimus dorsi, pectoralis major, teres major, deltoid, triceps, and trapezius. Certain intrinsic factors associated with the donor tissue that must be respected involve length of the muscle and tendon unit, line of action relative to joint rotation, and amplitude of the generated force [41].

It is imperative that patient expectations are appropriately clarified preoperatively, and anyone that undergoes this type of procedure must understand its magnitude and the rigors behind the postoperative physical therapy. Advanced glenohumeral arthritis must be excluded, and the ideal candidate will have symptoms related to weakness and impaired active motion. Manuel laborers with irreparable rotator cuff tears who require strength to resume typical occupational task are often cited as the archetypal patient population [1].

Latissimus Dorsi Transfer

Initially proposed by Gerber in 1988, the latissimus dorsi provides appropriate excursion for the treatment of external rotation deficits in posterosuperior rotator cuff tears [42]. The tendon is thus converted to a humeral head depressor through its vertical orientation and an external rotator via its new relative insertion in the humeral head [41]. A functioning deltoid is a prerequisite for a successful result, and ideally the tendon of the subscapularis must also be intact to provide a balanced force couple in the coronal plane [8]. Gerber was also able to demonstrate technical feasibility and early therapeutic efficacy through cadaveric and clinical studies [43].

Gerber [44] later corroborated his results with long-term studies on the value of latissimus transfers for irreparable posterosuperior rotator cuff tears. He evaluated 63 patients at a mean follow-up of 53 months and demonstrated reliably durable results. Average subjective shoulder value scores increase 35 % postoperatively, and mean Constant scores also increased 20 % from their preoperative value. Furthermore, pain, forward flexion, abduction, external rotation, and strength all improved with statistical significance. Positive results have also been shown by numerous authors in the setting of failed rotator cuff repair [45, 46].

To further evaluate the inherent value and appropriate timing of a proposed latissimus transfer, Warner and Parsons compared outcomes in patients who underwent tendon transfer as a primary reconstruction option to those who underwent transfer for salvage reconstruction [8]. Although patient numbers were small (16 patients in the primary group and 6 patients in the salvage reconstruction group), important findings were noted. At a mean follow-up of 2 years, relative gain of forward flexion was 60° versus 43°, in the primary and salvage reconstruction groups, respectively. The primary group also demonstrated greater improvement in relative Constant score after tendon transfer.

Technical considerations, when performing the transfer, include cognizance of the radial and axillary nerve and their relationship to known anatomic landmarks [47]. Iannotti et al. have identified important patient characteristics that portend a poor outcome – female sex, poor preoperative glenohumeral function, and generalized muscle weakness [48]. Recent modifications to the transfer technique have also been published that include harvesting a small piece of bone with the tendon [49], utilization of a single incision [50], and minimally invasive approaches [51]. None have demonstrated superior clinical results to Gerber's initial description [9].

Pectoralis Major Transfer

Transfer of the pectoralis major tendon remains a viable treatment option for those patients who have sustained an irreparable tear of the anterosuperior rotator cuff with concomitant deficits in internal rotation power. Recently, much attention has been paid to the line of pull of the pectoralis major, and consequently, modifications of the original technique have been made to improve the vector and fulcrum over which the transferred tendon occurs. Wirth and Rockwood initially reported satisfactory results in 10/13 patients who underwent pectoralis transfer above the coracoid [52]. However, more recent biomechanical and clinical data has suggested an advantage to isolated sternal head transfer, in a subcoracoid fashion, of the pectoralis major tendon [53, 54]. The sternal head can be passed beneath the clavicular head, so that the latter may act as a fulcrum, thus allowing for a more anatomic recreation of the force couple of the torn subscapularis.

Elhassaan et al. reported on 11 patients in whom the sternal head subcoracoid technique was utilized for the treatment of irreparable subscapularis tears. Improvement in pain scores occurred in 7/11 patients at a minimum of 2 years follow-up. Functional improvement also occurred by measurement of postoperative Constant and subjective shoulder scores [53]. Resch et al. were able to demonstrate comparable results in an older cohort (mean age 65 years), utilizing a similar surgical technique. Good to excellent outcomes were reported in 9/12 patients, and mean Constant scores improved from 26.9 to 67.1 points postoperatively. All 12 tendon transfers demonstrated successful healing, as determined by ultrasound examination, at a mean final follow-up of 28 months [54]. In a larger series Jost et al were able to validate reliable results that

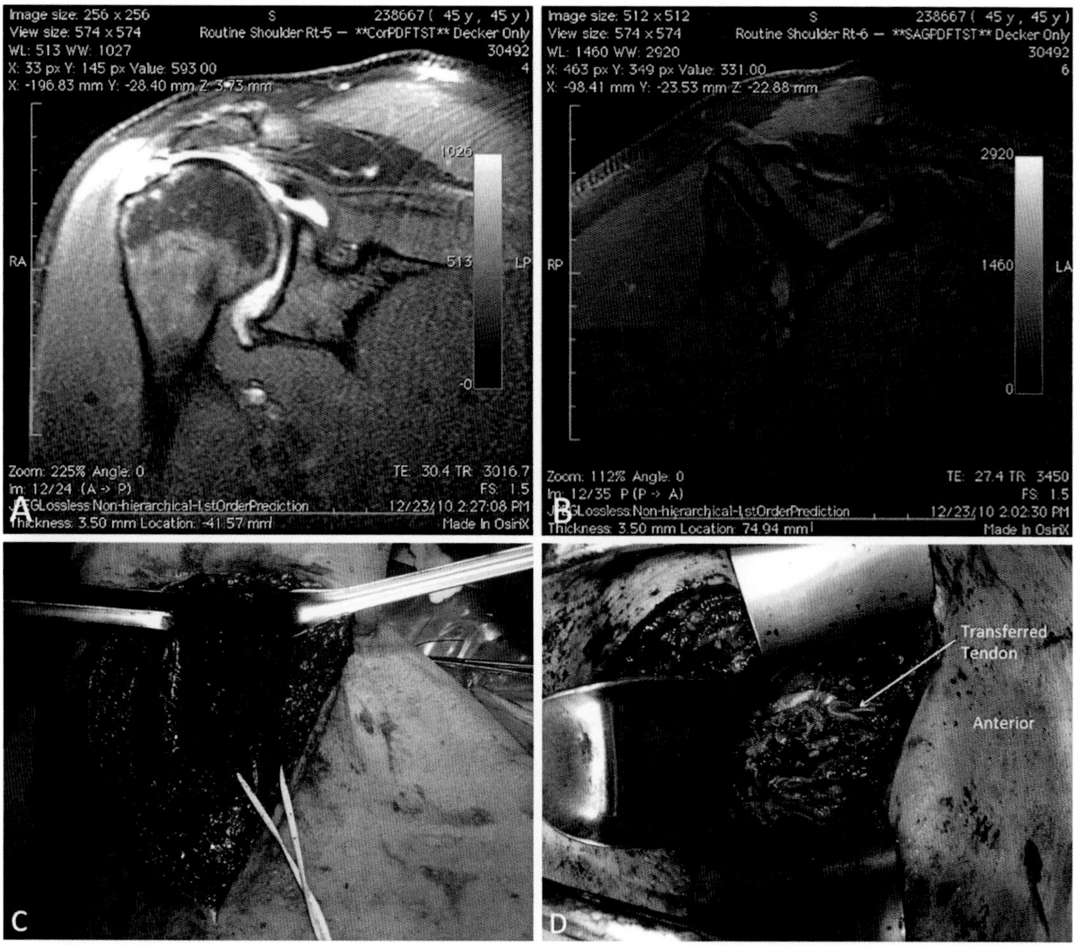

Fig. 11.2 Patient is a 45-year-old male with a 2-year history of pain and weakness. He has undergone two previous arthroscopic rotator cuff repairs. He is able to elevate his arm above his head, but it is weak particularly in external rotation. Coronal MRI shows a large rotator cuff tear with humeral head elevation (**a**). Sagittal MRI shows severe fatty infiltration of his infraspinatus and moderate infiltration of his supraspinatus (**b**). Patient elected to undergo latissimus dorsi transfer through a two-incision approach (**c**, **d**). A xenograft was used to augment the thin latissimus dorsi tendon prior to repair (**d**). Eighteen months following the surgery, the patient has improved strength and minimal pain

were not dependent on the routing of the transferred tendon, and 24 of 30 patients demonstrated satisfactory results at a final follow-up of 32 months. Mean relative Constant scores improved by 23 %. Markedly better outcomes were noted in those patients being treated for isolated irreparable subscapularis tears [55].

Author's Preferred Use of Tendon Transfers

The indications for tendon transfers are narrow. Ideal patients for latissimus dorsi transfer are men under the age of 50, whose chief complaint is weakness. These patients must still maintain the ability to elevate to horizontal and have an intact subscapularis with minimal underlying glenohumeral osteoarthritis. When examining a potential candidate, the examiner can help the patient elevate their arms with two fingers. This additional assistance roughly predicts what a latissimus dorsi transfer can provide. A two-incision technique is utilized and the latissimus dorsi alone is transferred to the greater tuberosity. Often, the tendon is reinforced with a tissue scaffold since it is relatively thin (Fig. 11.2). Recently, the author has been inserting the transferred tendon to the greater tuberosity arthroscopically by using knotless suture anchors. This avoids the added morbidity of deltoid takedown and repair.

Pectoralis major transfers are reserved for patients with isolated irreparable subscapularis ruptures. The sternal head is transferred under the conjoint tendon and attached to the lesser tuberosity. If the patients have undergone previous surgery in the region, then a hand surgeon is utilized to free the axillary and musculocutaneous nerves prior to transfer.

Both transfers require a long rehabilitation. The first 6 weeks are dedicated to healing so a sling is used and gentle pendulum exercises are started. From 6 to 12 weeks, passive range of motion is achieved. At 12 weeks, strengthening starts and patients are given a biofeedback machine to help retrain the transferred muscles. Patients are told that improvements will continue to be made up to a year out from surgery.

Scaffold Devices

Strategies that involve a tissue engineering approach, to address the problems associated with the unpredictable results following repair of massive rotator cuff tears, have received renewed interest, both bench side and in the clinical arena. Specifically, many studies have investigated the utility of scaffold devices to ensure improved rotator cuff healing. Scaffolds have the unique ability to improve both the mechanical and biologic environment after rotator cuff surgery. Theoretically they can "off-load" repair sites and possibly allow for efficient cellular ingrowth and proliferation [56]. Many devices are currently approved by the US Food and Drug Administration (FDA) for augmentation of rotator cuff repair and can be broadly categorized into extracellular matrix (ECM) devices, synthetic devices, and hybrid devices. Presently, no device is approved for bridging the gap of an irreparable rotator cuff repair, and this use remains off-label [3]. ECM-derived devices offer a distinct biologic advantage to the repair milieu site, whereas synthetic devices will maintain mechanical properties over time and can stabilize repairs while healing occurs [57].

Trials evaluating the results of ECM scaffolds as a bridging interpositional device for rotator cuff repair have demonstrated varying results [58, 59]. Soler et al. investigated the use of porcine dermal collagen implants in four patients at 3–6 months follow-up. The cohort age range was 71–82 years old, and graft disintegration, accompanied by an inflammatory reaction, was noted in all patients [58]. Authors of a similar study showed more promising results, utilizing an analogous construct for the bridging of a rotator cuff defect, in ten patients that were followed for 3–5 years. Mean Constant scores improved from 42 to 62 at final follow-up, while pain, abduction power, and range of motion were all significantly improved. Postoperative ultrasound demonstrated that 8/10 grafts were intact, and no patients sustained any significant adverse events [59]. Dermis-based patches have also been studied for salvage reconstruction of irreparable rotator cuff tears. Bond et al. reviewed 16 patients treated with dermal allograft for contracted immobile rotator cuff tears. At a mean follow-up of 2 years, patients experienced statistically improved measurements in pain level, forward flexion, and external rotation strength. Full incorporation of the graft occurred in 13/16 patients, as measured on MRI, and Constant scores improved a total of 30 points [60].

Author's Preferred Use of Scaffolds

At this time, scaffolds or patches are not routinely used. There is typically enough tissue to adequately perform a margin convergence repair and thus cover the humeral head with native tissue. The addition of synthetic or foreign material is thought to do little to augment these nonanatomic repairs. Scaffolds are not strong enough to serve as a bridging device.

Arthroplasty

Glenohumeral joint replacement may often be the appropriate primary or salvage option in patients with irreparable rotator cuff tears.

Patients who may benefit most from the various arthroplasty options are those patients who have the underlying diagnosis of rotator cuff tear arthropathy, although reliable preliminary results have also been obtained in patients without concomitant arthritis [61].

Hemiarthroplasty

Replacement of the humeral head is best reserved for patients who have maintained balanced mechanics of the glenohumeral joint – preserved coronal plane force couple (intact subscapularis) and continue to have the ability to elevate their affected arm [2]. Anterosuperior escape of the humeral head is generally considered a contraindication to humeral head replacement in patient with cuff tear arthropathy (CTA) [41].

Functional results following hemiarthroplasty for the diagnosis of CTA have been mixed. Sanchez-Sotelo showed successful results in only 67 % of cases at a mean of 5 years follow-up [62]. Active elevation improved 20° postoperatively; however, no strength differences were noted in abduction or flexion. Field et al. reviewed the results of hemiarthroplasty for treatment of CTA in 16 patients followed for a mean of 33 months. Overall results were encouraging, with 63 % of patients displaying satisfactory results. Patients who had undergone a previous acromioplasty were more prone to postoperative anterosuperior escape [63]. These results were confirmed by Zuckerman et al. who retrospectively reviewed 15 cases of humeral head replacement for the diagnosis of CTA. All patients demonstrated improved ability to perform ADLs and 13/15 patients expressed overall satisfaction with their result. Functionally patients exhibited improved forward flexion, external rotation, and UCLA scores.

Reverse Shoulder Arthroplasty (RSA)

Patients with true pseudoparalysis on exam are ideal candidates for an RSA prosthesis, in the setting of massive irreparable rotator cuff tears, with or without underlying osteoarthritis. Recent literature out of France supports the use of the RSA in the absence of arthritis [61]. Wall and colleagues demonstrated a Constant score improvement of 36 points, in 34 such patients. On specific subscales pain improved 8 points, activity level 10 points, mobility 12 points, and strength 6 points. Range of motion improvements were the most dramatic, showing increased elevation from 94° to 143°.

Many authors at multiple institutions have confirmed successful results of the RSA, when used for rotator cuff tear arthropathy. Wener et al. reported on 17 consecutive patients, who were followed for 38 months. Marked functional objective gains were noted, with an overall Constant score improvement of 35–72 points [64]. Active abduction increased from 39° to 84°, and forward flexion followed with a net gain of 60°. Frankle corroborated these results in 60 patients who were treated for CTA and later evaluated at a minimum of 2 years. The average ASES scores improved 34 points postoperatively, and active forward flexion improved from 55° to 105° [65].

It must be noted that short- and midterm results with the reverse prosthesis are promising; however, a substantial complication rate has been noted. Prosthetic survival rate at 8 years has been reported as 30 % [66]. Overall complication rates have been reported as high as 50 %, with 33 % of patients requiring a revision surgery [64].

Author's Preferred Use of Arthroplasty

Rare patients with advanced cuff tear arthropathy and the preserved ability to elevate are offered hemiarthroplasty. In these situations, every effort is made to preserve the CA arch and the subscapularis – two primary reasons why the patient may still be able to elevate their arm. With the exceptions of very large males, most hemiarthroplasties can be inserted through the superior rotator cuff defect without taking down the subscapularis with a deltopectoral incision. Rehabilitation is fairly rapid, with sling immobilization only until the wound is healed; then aggressive motion and strengthening are undertaken.

Patients with an irreparable rotator cuff tear and true pseudoparalysis are ideal candidates for a reverse shoulder arthroplasty, with or without concomitant arthritis (Fig. 11.3). A deltopectoral approach is used. The subscapularis is reattached

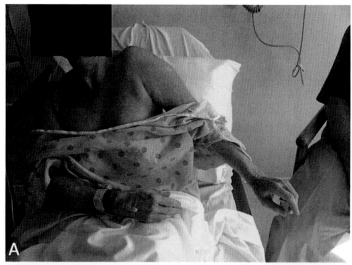

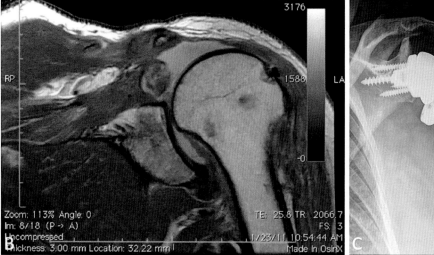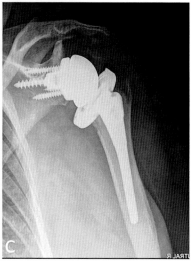

Fig. 11.3 Patient is a 69-year-old female with a 2-year history of shoulder pain and weakness. She has undergone one prior rotator cuff repair, but is now unable to elevate her arm above her head even after an injection with local anesthetic. She also has anterosuperior escape with attempts at elevation (**a**). MRI in the coronal plane shows a massive, retracted tear with humeral head elevation (**b**). Patient underwent reverse total shoulder arthroplasty (**c**). Three years after the procedure, she is pain free and able to elevate to 170°

if it is present and can be repaired tension free. Rehabilitation consists of sling immobilization for 2 weeks and then a rapid restoration of motion and strength. Therapists are informed not to force internal rotation, since these limitations are most often due to implant impingement and not soft tissue contracture.

Conclusion

The irreparable rotator cuff tear continues to present as a challenging treatment dilemma for orthopedic surgeons. A cadre of treatment options exists, and it is imperative that careful patient evaluation and management allow for an

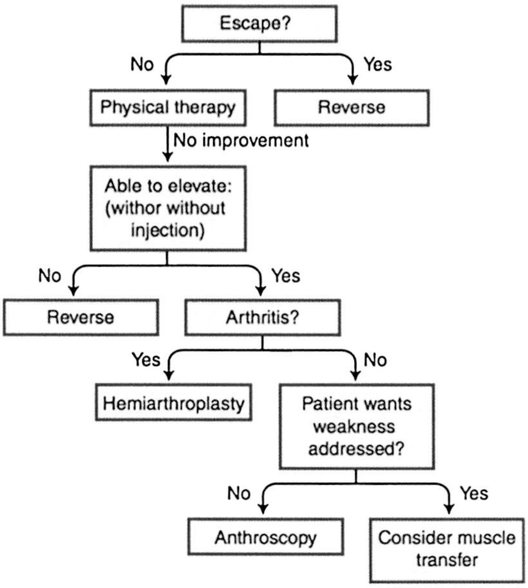

Fig. 11.4 Treatment algorithm for patients with irreparable rotator cuff tears (Reprinted with permission from Khair and Gulotta [2])

individualized plan based on symptoms and physical exam findings. The authors have previously proposed a reasonable and reproducible treatment algorithm that can be applied to patients with symptomatic irreparable rotator cuff tears (Fig. 11.4) [2].

In the absence of anterosuperior escape, physical therapy, with a focus on anterior deltoid strengthening, must be exhausted prior to undergoing any surgical intervention. Determination of the primary symptom and complaint of the patient is vital to a successful outcome in those patients who have failed physical therapy (or already have anterosuperior escape). Local anesthetic injection in the subacromial space can provide useful diagnostic and therapeutic value to discern true pseudoparalysis. Those patients who can actively elevate their arm are candidates for debridement, partial repair, biceps tenotomy, and possible SSN release. A latissimus transfer should then be considered in those patients who have the primary complaint of external rotation weakness with an intact subscapularis tendon. Arthritis, as demonstrated on plain radiographs, should be treated with an arthroplasty option that

is dictated by the mechanical state of the glenohumeral joint. Humeral head arthroplasty should be undertaken in those patients that continue to have ability to elevate their arm overhead, while reverse shoulder arthroplasty should be considered in those with pseudoparalysis.

References

1. Bedi A, Dines J, Warren RF, Dines D. Massive tears of the rotator cuff. J Bone Joint Surg Am. 2010;92: 1894–908.
2. Khair M, Gulotta LV. Treatment of irreparable rotator cuff tears. Curr Rev Musculoskelet Med. 2011;4:208–13.
3. Neri B, Chan K, Kwon Y. Management of massive and irreparable rotator cuff tears. J Shoulder Elbow Surg. 2009;18:808–18.
4. Cofield RH. Rotator cuff disease of the shoulder. J Bone Joint Surg Am. 1985;67:974–9.
5. Nobuhara K, Hata Y, Komai M. Surgical procedure and results of repair of massive tears of the rotator cuff. Clin Orthop Relat Res. 1994;(304):54–9.
6. Burkhart SS. Arthroscopic treatment of massive rotator cuff tears. Clinical results and biomechanical rationale. Clin Orthop Relat Res. 1991;267:45–56.
7. Gerber C, Fuchs B, Hodler J. The results of repair of massive tears of the rotator cuff. J Bone Joint Surg Am. 2000;82(4):505–15.
8. Warner JJ, Parsons IM. Latissimus dorsi tendon transfer: a comparative analysis of primary and salvage reconstruction of massive, irreparable rotator cuff tears. J Shoulder Elbow Surg. 2001;10(6):514–21.
9. Delaney R, Lin A, Warner JP. Nonarthroplasty options for the management of massive and irreparable rotator cuff tears. Clin Sports Med. 2012;31:727–48.
10. Burkhart SS. Arthroscopic treatment of massive rotator cuff tears. Clinical results and biomechanical rationale. Clin Orthop Relat Res. 1991;(267):45–56.
11. Sher JS, Uribe JW, Posada A, Murphy BJ, Zlatkin MB. Abnormal findings on magnetic resonance images of asymptomatic shoulders. J Bone Joint Surg Am. 1995;77:10–5.
12. Tempelhof S, Rupp S, Seil R. Age-related prevalence of rotator cuff tears in asymptomatic shoulders. J Shoulder Elbow Surg. 1999;8:296–9.
13. Boes MT, McCann PD, Dines DM. Diagnosis and management of massive rotator cuff tears: the surgeon's dilemma. Instr Course Lect. 2006;55:45–57.
14. Hertel R, Ballmer FT, Lombert SM, Gerber C. Lag signs in the diagnosis of rotator cuff rupture. J Shoulder Elbow Surg. 1996;5:307–13.
15. Walch G, Boulahia A, Calderone S, Robinson AH. The 'dropping' and 'hornblower's' signs in evaluation of rotator-cuff tears. J Bone Joint Surg Br. 1998;80:624–8.

16. Hamada K, Fukuda H, Mikasa M, Kobayashi Y. Roentgenographic findings in massive rotator cuff tears. A long-term observation. Clin Orthop Relat Res. 1990;(254):92–6.

17. Werner CM, Conrad SJ, Meyer DC, Keller A, Hodler J, Gerber C. Intermethod agreement and interobserver correlation of radiologic acromiohumeral distance measurements. J Shoulder Elbow Surg. 2008;17:237–40.

18. Iannotti JP, Zlatkin MB, Esterhai JL, Kressel HY, Dalinka MK, Spindler KP. Magnetic resonance imaging of the shoulder. Sensitivity, specificity, and predictive value. J Bone Joint Surg Am. 1991;73:17–29.

19. Harryman 2nd DT, Mack LA, Wang KY, Jackins SE, Richardson ML, Matsen 3rd FA. Repairs of the rotator cuff. Correlation of functional results with integrity of the cuff. J Bone Joint Surg Am. 1991;73:982–9.

20. Goutallier D, Postel JM, Bernageau J, Lavau L, Voisin MC. Fatty muscle degeneration in cuff ruptures. Pre- and postoperative evaluation by CT scan. Clin Orthop Relat Res. 1994;304:78–83.

21. Goutallier D, Postel JM, Gleyze P, Leguilloux P, Van Driessche S. Influence of cuff muscle fatty degeneration on anatomic and functional outcomes after simple suture of full-thickness tears. J Shoulder Elbow Surg. 2003;12:550–4.

22. Mellado JM, Calmet J, Olona M, Esteve C, Camins A, Pérez Del Palomar L, Giné J, Saurí A. Surgically repaired massive rotator cuff tears: MRI of tendon integrity, muscle fatty degeneration, and muscle atrophy correlated with intraoperative and clinical findings. AJR Am J Roentgenol. 2005;184:1456–63.

23. Hansen ML, Otis JC, Johnson JS, Cordasco FA, Craig EV, Warren RF. Biomechanics of massive rotator cuff tears: implications for treatment. J Bone Joint Surg Am. 2008;90:316–25.

24. DePalma AF. Surgical anatomy of the rotator cuff and the natural history of degenerative periarthritis. Surg Clin North Am. 1963;43:1507–20.

25. Ainsworth R. Physiotherapy rehabilitation in patients with massive, irreparable rotator cuff tears. Musculoskeletal Care. 2006;4:140–51.

26. Levy O, Mullett H, Roberts S, Copeland S. The role of anterior deltoid reeducation in patients with massive irreparable degenerative rotator cuff tears. J Shoulder Elbow Surg. 2008;17:863–70.

27. Fenlin Jr JM, Chase JM, Rushton SA, Frieman BG. Tuberoplasty: creation of an acromiohumeral articulation – a treatment option for massive, irreparable rotator cuff tears. J Shoulder Elbow Surg. 2002; 11:136–42.

28. Burkhart SS. Partial repair of massive rotator cuff tears: the evolution of a concept. Orthop Clin North Am. 1997;28:125–32.

29. Burkhart SS, Nottage WM, Ogilvie-Harris DJ, Kohn HS, Pachelli A. Partial repair of irreparable rotator cuff tears. Arthroscopy. 1994;10:363–70.

30. Duralde XA, Bair B. Massive rotator cuff tears: the result of partial rotator cuff repair. J Shoulder Elbow Surg. 2005;14:121–7.

31. Pagnani MJ, Deng XH, Warren RF, Torzilli PA, Altchek DW. Effect of lesions of the superior portion of the glenoid labrum on glenohumeral translation. J Bone Joint Surg Am. 1995;77:1003–110.

32. Pagnani MJ, Deng XH, Warren RF, Torzilli PA, O'Brien SJ. Role of the long head of the biceps brachii in glenohumeral stability: a biomechanical study in cadavera. J Shoulder Elbow Surg. 1996;5:255–62.

33. Yamaguchi K, Riew KD, Galatz LM, Syme JA, Neviaser RJ. Biceps activity during shoulder motion: an electromyographic analysis. Clin Orthop Relat Res. 1997;336:122–9.

34. Walch G, Edwards TB, Boulahia A, Nové-Josserand L, Neyton L, Szabo I. Arthroscopic tenotomy of the long head of the biceps in the treatment of rotator cuff tears: clinical and radiographic results of 307 cases. J Shoulder Elbow Surg. 2005;14(3):238–46.

35. Boileau P, Baque F, Valerio L, Ahrens P, Chuinard C, Trojani C. Isolated arthroscopic biceps tenotomy or tenodesis improves symptoms in patients with massive irreparable rotator cuff tears. J Bone Joint Surg Am. 2007;89(4):747–57.

36. Boykin RE, Friedman DJ, Zimmer ZR, Oaklander AL, Higgins LD, Warner JJ. Suprascapular neuropathy in a shoulder referral practice. J Shoulder Elbow Surg. 2011;20(6):983–8.

37. Lafosse L, Tomasi A, Corbett S, Baier G, Willems K, Gobezie R. Arthroscopic release of suprascapular nerve entrapment at the suprascapular notch: technique and preliminary results. Arthroscopy. 2007; 23(1):34–42.

38. Costouros JG, Porramatikul M, Lie DT, Warner JJ. Reversal of suprascapular neuropathy following arthroscopic repair of massive supraspinatus and infraspinatus rotator cuff tears. Arthroscopy. 2007; 23(11):1152–61.

39. Warner JP, Krushell RJ, Masquelet A, Gerber C. Anatomy and relationships of the suprascapular nerve: anatomical constraints to mobilization of the supraspinatus and infraspinatus muscles in the management of massive rotator-cuff tears. J Bone Joint Surg Am. 1992;74(1):36–45.

40. Mallon WJ, Wilson RJ, Basamania CJ. The association of suprascapular neuropathy with massive rotator cuff tears: a preliminary report. J Shoulder Elbow Surg. 2006;15(4):395–8.

41. Warner JJ. Management of massive irreparable rotator cuff tears: the role of tendon transfer. Instr Course Lect. 2001;50:63–71.

42. Gerber C, Vinh TS, Hertel R, Hess CW. Latissimus dorsi transfer for the treatment of massive tears of the rotator cuff. A preliminary report. Clin Orthop Relat Res. 1988;232:51–61.

43. Gerber C, Maquieira G, Espinosa N. Latissimus dorsi transfer for the treatment of irreparable rotator cuff tears. J Bone Joint Surg Am. 2006;88(1):113–20.

44. Gerber C. Latissimus dorsi transfer for the treatment of irreparable tears of the rotator cuff. Clin Orthop Relat Res. 1992;275:152–60.

45. Birmingham PM, Neviaser RJ. Outcome of latissimus dorsi transfer as a salvage procedure for failed rotator cuff repair with loss of elevation. J Shoulder Elbow Surg. 2008;17(6):871–4.

46. Miniaci A, MacLeod M. Transfer of the latissimus dorsi muscle after failed repair of a massive tear of the rotator cuff. A two to five-year review. J Bone Joint Surg Am. 1999;81(8):1120–7.

47. Morelli M, Nagamori J, Gilbart M, Miniaci A. Latissimus dorsi tendon transfer for massive irreparable cuff tears: an anatomic study. J Shoulder Elbow Surg. 2008;17(1):139–43.

48. Iannotti JP, Hennigan S, Herzog R, Kella S, Kelly M, Leggin B, Williams GR. Latissimus dorsi tendon transfer for irreparable posterosuperior rotator cuff tears. Factors affecting outcome. J Bone Joint Surg Am. 2006;88(2):342–8.

49. Moursy M, Forstner R, Koller H, Resch H, Tauber M. Latissimus dorsi tendon transfer for irreparable rotator cuff tears: a modified technique to improve tendon transfer integrity. J Bone Joint Surg Am. 2009;91(8):1924–31.

50. Habermeyer P, Magosch P, Rudolph T, Lichtenberg S, Liem D. Transfer of the tendon of latissimus dorsi for the treatment of massive tears of the rotator cuff: a new single-incision technique. J Bone Joint Surg Br. 2006;88(2):208–12.

51. Lehmann LJ, Mauerman E, Strube T, Laibacher K, Scharf HP. Modified minimally invasive latissimus dorsi transfer in the treatment of massive rotator cuff tears: a two-year follow-up of 26 consecutive patients. Int Orthop. 2010;34(3):377–83.

52. Wirth MA, Rockwood Jr CA. Operative treatment of irreparable rupture of the subscapularis. J Bone Joint Surg Am. 1997;79(5):722–31.

53. Elhassan B, Ozbaydar M, Massimini D, Diller D, Higgins L, Warner JJ. Transfer of pectoralis major for the treatment of irreparable tears of subscapularis: does it work? J Bone Joint Surg Br. 2008;90(8):1059–165.

54. Resch H, Povacz P, Ritter E, Matschi W. Transfer of the pectoralis major muscle for the treatment of irreparable rupture of the subscapularis tendon. J Bone Joint Surg Am. 2000;82(3):372–82.

55. Jost B, Puskas GJ, Lustenberger A, Gerber C. Outcome of pectoralis major transfer for the treatment of irreparable subscapularis tears. J Bone Joint Surg Am. 2003;85-A(10):1944–51.

56. Ricchetti E, Aurora A, Iannotti J, Derwin K. Scaffold devices for rotator cuff repair. J Shoulder Elbow Surg. 2012;21:251–65.

57. Encalada-Diaz I, Cole BJ, MacGillivray JD, Ruiz-Suarez M, Kercher JS, Friel NA, et al. Rotator cuff repair augmentation using a novel polycarbonate polyurethane patch: preliminary results at 12 months' follow-up. J Shoulder Elbow Surg. 2011;20:788–94.

58. Soler JA, Gidwani S, Curtis MJ. Early complications from the use of porcine dermal collagen implants (Permacol) as bridging constructs in the repair of massive rotator cuff tears. A report of 4 cases. Acta Orthop Belg. 2007;73:432–6.

59. Badhe SP, Lawrence TM, Smith FD, Lunn PG. An assessment of porcine dermal xenograft as an augmentation graft in the treatment of extensive rotator cuff tears. J Shoulder Elbow Surg. 2008;17:35S–9.

60. Bond JL, Dopirak RM, Higgins J, Burns J, Snyder SJ. Arthroscopic replacement of massive, irreparable rotator cuff tears using a Graft-Jacket allograft: technique and preliminary results. Arthroscopy. 2008;24:403–9.

61. Wall B, Nové-Josserand L, O'Connor DP, Edwards TB, Walch G. Reverse total shoulder arthroplasty: a review of results according to etiology. J Bone Joint Surg Am. 2007;89:1476–85.

62. Sanchez-Sotelo J, Cofield RH, Rowland CM. Shoulder hemiarthroplasty for glenohumeral arthritis associated with severe rotator cuff deficiency. J Bone Joint Surg Am. 2001;83-A(12):1814–22.

63. Field LD, Dines DM, Zabinski SJ, Warren RF. Hemiarthroplasty of the shoulder for rotator cuff arthropathy. J Shoulder Elbow Surg. 1997;6:18–23.

64. Werner CM, Steinmann PA, Gilbart M, Gerber C. Treatment of painful pseudoparesis due to irreparable rotator cuff dysfunction with the Delta III reverse-ball-and-socket total shoulder prosthesis. J Bone Joint Surg Am. 2005;87(7):1476–86.

65. Frankle M, Levy JC, Pupello D, Siegal S, Saleem A, Mighell M, Vasey M. The reverse shoulder prosthesis for glenohumeral arthritis associated with severe rotator cuff deficiency. A minimum two year follow-up study of sixty patients surgical technique. J Bone Joint Surg Am. 2006;88(Suppl 1 Pt 2):178–90.

66. Guery J, Favard L, Sirveaux F, Oudet D, Mole D, Walch G. Reverse total shoulder arthroplasty. Survivorship analysis of eighty replacements followed for five to ten years. J Bone Joint Surg Am. 2006;88:1742–7.

Index